It's All In Your Head!
The Gene That Stumped
The Doctors

It's All In Your Head! The Gene That Stumped The Doctors

TRUE ACCOUNT OF A SURVIVOR'S STORY, WHICH DATES BACK 50+ YEARS, AND HOW DNA SAVED HER LIFE

Kittye Sharron

kittyesharron1@gmail.com
www.facebook.com/kittyesharron
www.kittyesharron.com

Copyright © 2017 Kittye Sharron
All rights reserved.

ISBN: 1544974345
ISBN 13: 9781544974347

Table of Contents

Foreword vii
Introduction. xi
Prologue. xiii

Chapter 1	Ready or Not	1
Chapter 2	The Start of a New Life	6
Chapter 3	How Poor was Poor?	35
Chapter 4	Oh What a Life!.	57
Chapter 5	My Million Dollar Bill.	73
Chapter 6	Our World Turns Upside Down.	82
Chapter 7	Breast Cancer, The Best Thing That Ever Happened to Me!	91
Chapter 8	Microscopic No More	101
Chapter 9	My Little Girl Book	104
Chapter 10	Devotions at 3	108
Chapter 11	My Red Pen Ministry	114
Chapter 12	Dancing with My Husband	117

Chapter 13	Parting Words	124
Chapter 14	Let's Talk Hair & Gray & Izzy!	132
Chapter 15	Pictures & Years of Hairstyles	139
	Epilogue (2017)	143
	Acknowledgements	147
	About the Author.	153

Foreword

"KITTYE'S STORY IS AN IMPORTANT *one to tell. Without her resilience and determination, an entire family and its future generations may never have known about the rare condition for which they are at risk.*

Hereditary Paraganglioma-Pheochromocytoma Syndrome (PGL-PCC) is estimated to occur in 1 in 300,000 to 1 in one million people. After her diagnosis, Kittye gladly participated in our annual "Cancer Genetics" presentation given to 3rd year medical students. We later received many positive reviews of her presentation, and students commented on how much they appreciated Kittye's willingness to share her story. If these students learned anything from Kittye, it is that a good doctor listens to his/her patients.

We are honored to have had the opportunity to work with Kittye, and now her family members as they come for their own genetics consult."

MARY C. MOBLEY, MEd, MS, CGC

Dedication

Having a sister is like having a mother,
You could look the world over and never find another.
When I left home I never thought I'd miss
That bratty little kid, my little sis.
When we were kids, such a pest she could be,
She'd go to extremes just to get a rise out of me.
Sometimes she made me a nervous wreck
And the things she did, I could have wrung her neck!
There were times I thought she hated me
But never could she see,
That all I wanted was to be left alone
When I yelled at her in that mean, harsh tone.
When I walked down that aisle to be married,
I remember the tears her little eyes carried.
And of marriage now is what she's talking
So pretty soon, down that same aisle she'll be walking.
It's enough to make you cry

Kittye Sharron

*And in a way, it's like saying goodbye.
But what I'll be doing is saying hello
To that big little girl whom I've always loved so.
Yes, I dedicate this to you, little sis
From the bottom of my heart and sealed with a kiss.
Thank you so much for being in my life,
But God help Ernie when you become his wife!*
(Written by: Kittye Sharron, AKA Amy Kayleen, for her sister, AKA Robyn Louise,; given in a card at her bridal shower in 1972.)

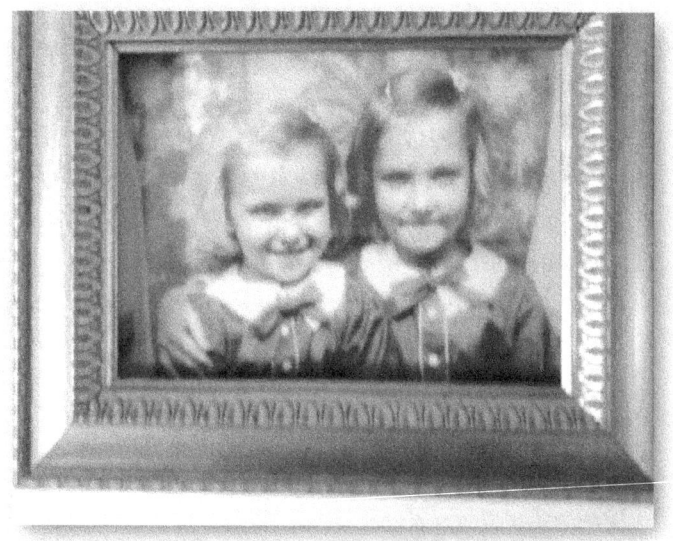

Picture above was made in 1954: AKA Robyn Louise (4) and AKA Amy Kayleen (6).

Introduction

"Oh no...how will I ever again be able to fix my hair?"

Now even though this book is not about fixing hair that was my first response when I fractured my left arm. Accidentally, I had tripped on the leg of a chair, causing me to lose my balance and fall onto the floor.

I've become known for the uniqueness of my hairstyle, which is featured on the front cover of this book. There is even a "how-to-do-it-yourself" video on my YouTube channel; also on my website. The last two chapters of this book will tell you how to get there, and will provide step-by-step instructions for achieving the look of the hairstyle, along with tips for greater enhancement.

It's no wonder I responded the way I did when fracturing my arm, since from the beginning of my time, hair had always been important to me. Even when we were just little girls, my mother used to spend countless hours putting my sister's and my hair in, what she called, finger curls. We hated it then, but looking back now, I'm so happy for those memories and pictures of our head shots. (Like the ones shown here; others are throughout the book.)

I certainly was thankful the fracture hadn't been in my right arm. In order to look presentable, with my good arm I was still able to, at least, anchor a few combs and clips on each side of my head. The orthopedic specialist said it would take 6 to 8 weeks, or longer, to heal; and he was right.

I've got too many things to do; I don't have time for this! Sometimes it's good to experience moments like those just to reflect on where life has been. *Looking back now, I can see,* I've been in many worse predicaments and, as you are about to discover, I had more in me than just a head of hair.

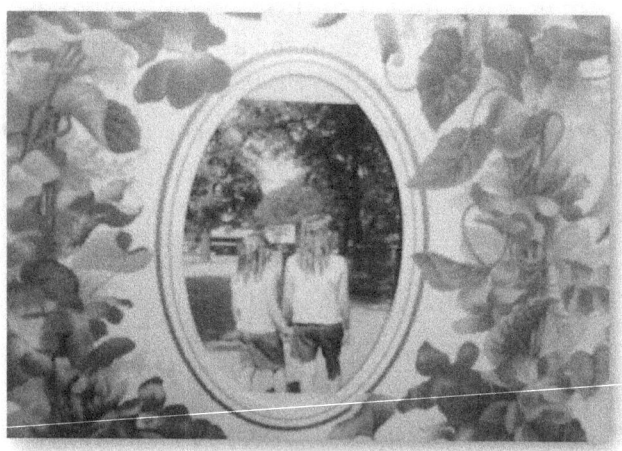

"Even when we were just little girls, my mother used to spend countless hours putting my sister's and my hair in, what she called, finger curls. We hated it then, but looking back now, I'm so happy for those memories and pictures of our head shots." (AKA Robyn Louise & Amy Kayleen.) **Quote by Kittye Sharron**

Prologue

"I was so hot that I slept in a bathtub full of cold water, every night, for six and a half years. In the middle of winter, I sat outside on the doorstep wearing only a sleeveless top and Bermuda shorts; I watched the snow melt as it fell on my bare skin."

QUOTE BY KITTYE SHARRON (*AKA AMY KAYLEEN.)

THE SECRET I WAS HIDING for 45+ years began to consume me. *(Sexually abused when 8 years old. Details of being attacked by a pedophile in 1956 are detailed in my first published book, "The Longest Letter: Incredible Hope.")* Even though many times I had tried to tell the story of the molestation, I could never get the words out, not even to my mother or my sister. *It was so horrible, so humiliating, even God would not understand!*

*One doesn't have a vocabulary to describe things of a sexual nature when only 8 years old; that's why 45+ years later, when the shame of it all became physical pain, I became Amy Kayleen and wrote about it. Assuming a different name after all those years allowed me the freedom to explain what had actually happened to me; once I wrote as Amy Kayleen, I was able to share it. *Therefore, as my writings unfold, I'll remain Amy Kayleen.*

> **Excerpt from the Longest Letter: Incredible Hope:**
> *"I was just a little girl from Arkansas who answered to the name of Amy Kayleen. My family was very poor, but I didn't know that then. I was with my parents; safe, content; until, at a tender age, violence, alcohol and abuse came into my life. Two things happened when I was 8 years old."*

Prior to that, I was just sure I could have been a great dancer but those dreams were quickly dashed when I was in first grade. My classmate had invited me to go with her after school and watch her perform at a dance recital. I was all of 6 years old, it was my lifelong dream, *and of course I'll go!* It didn't occur to me that the elderly woman with whom we were staying at the time would worry when I didn't arrive home right after school.

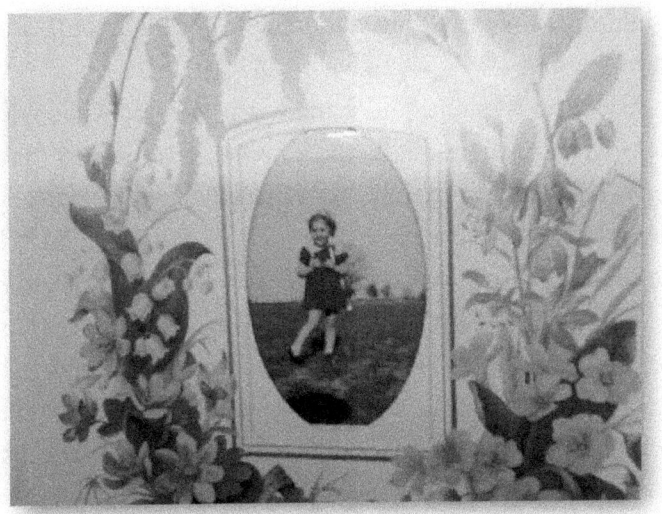

The dancer in little girl me. (AKA Amy Kayleen.)

It was dark when I did return, "Where have you been? You've been where? Shame on you!" I was sent to bed early. From the bedroom, I could hear my little sister, Robyn, say, "Can I have her cookie?"

Of course, it wasn't that dancing was wrong; it was the fact that I hadn't informed anyone of where I was, but I didn't know that then, which only fueled resentment and rebellion. I had just been watching someone else fulfill my own dreams which, obviously, would never come to fruition. Besides, there was no way I'd be able to have a cute little dance costume. My mother barely had enough money to provide us with mere essentials, let alone anything extra. Since my parents' separation, Mother had to do everything on her own; my father offered no help and had stopped coming to see us.

My sister, Robyn, and I made the best of what we had (i.e. using a rock for chalk and drawing a hopscotch pattern on the sidewalk; or making for ourselves a game whereby we looked through every page of an old Sears catalog and chose one of everything we hoped someday we'd have.) Someone had given us a pair of roller skates, which we took turns using, until we lost the skate key. After that we couldn't keep them on our feet. *That was long before the days of roller blades.*

Robyn and I used to have a lot of sore throats and, when I was seven, she was five, we had to have our tonsils removed. *I'm pretty sure it was our stay in the hospital that time that prompted the ruling requiring all patients to wear wrist bands while confined.*

We looked so much alike and people had a hard time telling us apart. An antibiotic shot was necessary prior to surgery and since I was the oldest, I was given the first shot. Then the nurse went out of the room, at which time Robyn and I decided to switch beds. When the nurse returned to give the next shot, I had an awful time convincing her that I had already had my shot. "Robyn Louise, you dang well better tell her you haven't had yours yet!"

Finally, the nurse figured it out and gave Robyn her shot. *Nobody at that time knew we shared more than a hospital room.*

Robyn was there with me a year later on that horrible night when that awful thing happened to me at 8 years old.

Even though she had been in the same room, she was asleep and thankfully did not witness it. When it was over, the 'little girl' in me reasoned it had been a bad dream, *"I will tell nobody, not ever!"*

From then on, I was angry. I had begun to feel like a throw away and did not view myself worthy of love. A few years after the molestation, toward the end of the 50's, my mother, my sister and I, (Robyn and me clutching our favorite dolls,) moved, with the clothes on our backs, via the Greyhound bus, from Arkansas to Michigan. (Before we left, Mother paid to have some of our other things, and the rest of our dolls, shipped to Michigan.) That's where my grandmother and grandfather (whom we called Mama and Nanny); uncles and two cousins were living. At least we would be nearer to Mother's side of the family. Mother remarried; my stepfather was very good to us.

We went to church once or twice a year but it wasn't consistent; my mother still had to work many weekends. Just prior to becoming a teenager I went to a weeklong vacation bible school and I remember hearing about the Lord, but there was a problem…the definition I had given myself lingered even after I walked the aisle and professed Jesus as my Savior. *I'm worthless! Damaged is no good!*

Because none of my ways changed, I stayed the same. As a result, I became a bitter, rebellious teenager and, more often than not, gave in to peer pressure and walked in the ways of the world. My focus was on self and what would please me. I thought nothing of skipping school whenever the opportunity presented itself. I also had a tendency toward foul language, and any idea hinting at trouble sounded good to me.

During the summer when I was sixteen, I enrolled at the Cosmetology school and took full time classes; thinking I might like to fix hair someday, *when I have a little girl!* When at home, in order for me to practice cutting hair, I used our dog. That stopped after I gave him a lion-cut; he was too embarrassed to go outside. My sister and her friend, Izzy, were happy to have me experiment on their hair; that is until I gave Izzy a hairstyle that, till this day, she's never forgotten! *(There is more about that memorable event in Chapter 14.)*

I continued my beauty school studies during 10th and 11th grades, completing the 1,500 required hours by attending evening and Saturday classes. It was during that time I began secretly smoking *(obviously, not one of my better decisions, but after all, isn't that what adults do?)*

In high school the only subjects in which I excelled were Shorthand and Typing so my mind often teetered on becoming a secretary versus a beautician, whatever it would take to just get out on my own.

At that time, the only goals I had in my life were to *hurry up* and graduate from high school, *hurry up* and get married, *hurry up* and be a wife, *hurry up* and have kids, just be a mother, and go to church … unable to slow down, *just hurry*, then *hurry* and *hurry* some more. All my life, there seemed to be this driving force within me which made me feel agitated, furious at times; less than peaceful. Even as a little girl, I often had debilitating headaches and was hyper, but tired. It didn't feel right, but I didn't know why or what to do about it.

Yes, I wanted to get married, have children and go to church! I figured happiness would just come. *I'll never get a divorce!* So, as soon as I barely got that high school diploma, the following month, August, 1966, I got married to a man in the military who was stationed abroad and periodically home on leaves. I remained in the states and worked as a secretary at a real estate office.

Two years later, in 1968, the first of my three sons was born, it surely was a surprise. You see, it was long before the days of ultrasound and finding out beforehand your baby's gender. I had just figured all along it would be a girl; no thought had entered my mind that it would be anything else.

"It's a boy? A boy! Are you sure? Count his fingers and toes and whatever else; is he all there?"

Oh my goodness, I don't know anything about little boys, there must be some mistake! I was supposed to have a girl!

One look at him, I was smitten, and I wouldn't have traded him for any girl; he was perfect, 7 pounds, 19 ½ inches long, and a head full of dark hair. (The doctor had to perform a short minor procedure, nothing serious, whereby he clipped a little strand of tissue under my son's tongue so he wouldn't have any trouble breastfeeding, which presented no lasting problems.) After my son was born, the doctor said he would probably be the biggest baby I would ever have. *Good thing, because I only weighed a little over 100 pounds my own self, and that was if I was sopping wet!*

I asked my mother, "Is he the most beautiful baby in the world or am I just biased?"

My mother's response regarding her first grandchild, "You'll have to ask someone besides me, I'm biased, too! I want him to call me Nana!"

What a glorious day that February 9th, 1968 had been. I had a son of whom I was so proud.

Two things occurred the following day. First, my father, while drinking, got himself into some kind of trouble with the law in a little town in Arkansas where he lived with his second wife and two year old son. Though unclear as to what, it landed him in the county jail which is where he died a few days later. The autopsy had indicated heart attack; he was only 42 years old. (There were suspicious circumstances, *and still are to this day*, we never did get all the answers. However, one thing was clear…while in jail, he had been beaten so badly that his eyeball was out of its socket and he was left to die in his cell. I swore to avenge my father's murder no matter how long it took; but nothing was going to bring my dad back to life. He had been a good man but, like many of us, made some bad decisions.)

Because I was in Michigan, still in the hospital, I didn't get to go to his funeral. Though miles and circumstances had separated us for many years, I still loved him and it hurt my heart that I was unable to pay my respects, or say my goodbyes. I had lost my maternal grandfather, Nanny, just two months prior; my emotions were wreaking havoc with me. *I can't even imagine what my dad's widow felt, since her two year old son, my half-brother, would also grow up without a father.* (Nobody knew at the time, but a decade later, the little guy would also lose his mother to death.)

The second thing that happened was that I started perspiring; not just under my arms, but all over my body. I was miserable even though it was a frigid February in Michigan, but not to me! I was so hot that when I would sleep on the bed a wet outline of my body would be there when I awoke. If cold, one can put on extra clothing, but when it seems as though you are burning up from the inside, you can't take off your skin! (Not that you would want to.) To get relief, I slept in a bathtub full of cold water! In the middle of winter, wearing only a sleeveless blouse and a pair of Bermuda shorts, I sat on the outside doorstep and watched the snow melt as it fell on my bare skin. Perspiration would drip from my head. I kept my hair short for comfort. I had stopped working a month prior to my son's birth to become a stay at home mother; which turned out to be a good thing, since it was uncomfortable to wear much clothing.

"God, can you help me?" I called out as if I was a 'little girl' again, scared yet seeking answers or solutions to something for which I had no control. It didn't matter how much water I drank; I was thirsty all the time, and hot, oh I was hot! It felt as though the top of my head was about to explode and spew out hot lava.

I began going to doctor after doctor looking for answers, to no avail. They would run tests and prescribe all kinds of medications, but the final diagnosis was always the same. "It's all in your head; nothing medically wrong!"

Wait a minute, do they think I'm crazy? Do I look crazy to you? Don't answer that! Maybe I was crazy! After all, I did set a haystack on fire once when I was about 10 years old. I had only been trying to learn how to smoke and got bored because I didn't know that in order to have smoke come out of my mouth I'd have to suck on the cigarette. The haystack behind which I was hiding caused me to think, "I wonder if hay will burn?" So, with a lit match…"Whoosh!" *Sure does! I think that's where the term originated, "Going up in smoke".*

Often I found myself thinking back to days of long ago and trying to figure out if there was anything I could have done differently in order to change what I was dealing with in the present. *Something is wrong with me, I'm not crazy!*

I mean, I come from good stock. My maternal grandparents were born and raised in the good state of Mississippi; even my mother was born there. They had moved to Arkansas and that's where my mother and father had met and married. My father was from a very big family and, according to my paternal grandmother, he had also perspired profusely. *Could this have anything to do with my dilemma?* I searched my memory to recall those discussions we had while sitting on her squeaky porch swing so many years ago. She said from early on my dad was always hot. When he was just a boy she would watch for him to come in from helping my grandfather in the field; invariably, he would be dripping with sweat as he ran to the house where she would be waiting at the door with a cold glass of water to give him. She made mention, that prior to his marrying my mother he was in the Army but, he had passed his physical with flying colors. Even with that information, I still had no answers as to what was causing me to be so hot.

I kept praying and asking the Lord to heal me; I knew something wasn't right. That went on for six and a half long years, during which time, even though my blood pressure remained high and I had two 1st trimester miscarriages, I gave birth two more times.

My 2nd beautiful son was born on June 19th, 1970, and weighed 10 pounds 8 oz... I suffered convulsions right after the birth. He was so big, and I so little, the doctor had to use forceps to bring him into the world. *Hey, big little guy, whatever happened to the prediction? You weren't supposed to be over 7 pounds!* Bless his little heart; his precious head and beautiful face were bruised from the forceps. But he was perfect in my eyes, and, in spite of the black and blue marks, he looked so healthy, and had a head full of thick, blonde hair. I was told that when he turned two he would need corrective surgery for a hypospadias (*a birth defect in which the urethra, the tube through which urine travels from the bladder to outside the body, wasn't properly developed.*) Too, he had a minor medical condition called jaundice (*a yellowing of the skin and eyes caused by too much bilirubin in the blood.*) The jaundice cleared up after a few days and he was allowed to go home. (*Bilirubin is an orange-yellow pigment, which is made naturally in the body when old red blood cells are broken down. After circulating in the blood, bilirubin then travels to the liver where it's excreted into the bile duct and stored in the gallbladder. If the body does not adequately remove it, and it becomes too high, liver damage can occur.*)

My labor had to be induced two weeks before the due date with my 3rd son. Otherwise, according to my doctor, the birth weight would have been over 13 pounds... *Nothing over 7 pounds, huh?!* My youngest son, after another natural delivery, was born on February 25th, 1973. When he was delivered, he ended up weighing 9 pounds 12 oz., after which time, I still only weighed in at a little over a 100 pounds. During the delivery, I lost so much blood, I had to have a blood transfusion. Of course, he too, was absolutely gorgeous with a head full of thick, black hair. Like his brother before him, he also had newborn jaundice which did not clear up on its own. Tiny shields were placed over his eyes and he was put under the bilirubin light (a type of fluorescent light which eliminates bilirubin from the blood) for a few days, which did, in fact, clear it up and he was allowed to go home.

During all that time, I continued to perspire profusely and experienced extreme fatigue, fits of rage, and oftentimes excruciating headaches. Over the course of 6 ½ years, I went to a total of 21 different doctors, each concluding I had a mental condition; other than high blood pressure, nothing was medically wrong. *I'd rather be anywhere than in a doctor's office! What should I do? Doesn't anyone know what I'm going through; anybody care? Sure, I know I'm not the sharpest tack in the box and, even though it was by the skin of my teeth, I did get through school. Yes, I know; I really do know that I should have paid more attention in Biology so I would be able to explain what is going on in my body!* Truth be known, the doctors just about had me convinced that I was ready for the loony bin!

GAZE INTO THE EYES
Gaze into the eyes of a person like me.
Erase the tears, what do you see?
Do you see confusion of life's mysteries?
Look into them, you might see me!
Totally in the dark at what it's all about,
But so much afraid
Someday I might find out!
(Written by: Kittye Sharron in the 1970's)

CHAPTER 1

Ready or Not

FINALLY, IN 1974, I STUMBLED upon a new doctor in town. He was a dermatologist who had just graduated from medical school and started his new practice in Muskegon, where I lived. The first day I went to see him, the parking lot next to his office was almost empty and it didn't take me long to realize that the few cars that were there most likely belonged to the office staff. There were no patients in his waiting room; not a good sign! *Any doctor who's worth anything always has a waiting room full of patients!*

When I went into the examining room, I began telling him my symptoms. He just kept looking at my hands and fingernails.

Then, raising his eyebrows, he stared directly into my eyes and with all seriousness said, "I think you have a tumor!"

With all seriousness, I quickly responded, "I think you're a quack! All the other doctors wanted to pump me full of medications and tell me it is all in my head. You want to cut me open!"

Devastated and angry, grabbing my purse, I got up to leave, at which time he said, "Just let me do one test on you; after all, what have you got to lose?"

He was right in more ways than one. Already feeling like I was losing my mind, I relented.

The test consisted of collecting my urine for two weeks. When the results came back, the doctor himself called me at home. Anyone who has faced a medical issue knows that when a doctor rings your telephone, it's never just a social call and what follows is not going to be good news.

Results were: Adrenaline, 7 times higher than normal!

The doctor stated he was certain I had a rare disease called Pheochromocytoma, and he was sure I had a tumor somewhere in my body which needed to come out. He instructed me to quickly arrange my personal life for an extended stay in the hospital and to report to his office as soon as possible, *today! My grandmother, Mama, always came to watch my kids whenever I was hospitalized; she was there this time, too.*

Once I was at his office, the doctor reached for my hand and pointed to my fingernails, stating that through my nail beds he could see evidence of a serious problem. He pointed to little purplish lines he called hematomas, under my fingernails, and said that I could die of a heart attack or stroke at any time!

By then, my brain had just about absorbed all it could handle and my level of comprehension was nonexistent, but he went on to explain that my catecholamine and the levels of metanephrines (*big words*) were abnormally elevated. More medical terms followed but my attention was focused on the fact that I needed surgery, and the big 'D' (*die*) word had been thrown in. My blood pressure was that of an 80 year old. **I was only 26 years old!**

Too much information! I don't have this book-learned stuff down! Again, I know that I should have paid more attention to biology and science. It was my sister who had the brains, not me; I was known for hiding my bad report card! I hated those subjects in school; just dissecting a frog in 10th grade caused me to have to go to the nurse's office! I can't wrap my mind around this! Can't you just spare me the details?

The dermatologist set up a team of doctors, all who thought the tumor might be on one of the two adrenal glands, since those were the only cases they knew of at that time. There were no CT scans nor MRIs back then. The only thing they could do was exploratory surgery. I was admitted to the hospital on August 5th, 1974. The night before my exploratory surgery was to begin, the surgeon came into my hospital room for a little talk.

He told me that very little was known about Pheochromocytoma. He said this type of tumor was usually hereditary, and that most people don't survive because by the time it is found, people are either in mental institutions or their graves. *Yeah, they go crazy trying to convince the doctors something is wrong, until it kills them!* He went on to say that even an autopsy typically would not reveal this rare condition. He informed me it would be a risky surgery, and said I had a 50/50 chance of surviving the operation. *Oh no, again, the big "D" word! I can't hear you, I don't want to listen to this!*

He said, "If anyone is going to make it it'll be you; you're a very persistent person and that may be the very thing that has saved your life." *You think? Yeah, but I'm not very brave!*

Then, he said something that changed the very course of my life, "If you have not made peace with your Maker, you might want to do so!" There was something about that big "M" word that really got my attention. The only time I remembered hearing that expression was when I was a just a little girl and we had gone to Mississippi to attend my maternal great-grandmother's funeral. The minister had said, "She has gone to meet her Maker…"

What? Am I really going to die? Surely, I'm not ready to meet my Maker, I'm not even 30 years old and besides, I'm not very good at this praying thing! Is there anybody else out there?

I watched the doctor walk out of my room. I swallowed the lump in my throat and, after I passed the time away by counting every dot on the ceiling, tears flooded my eyes. I thought about my dear children. I closed the door and turned off the light. Then, I got down on my knees on that cold, hard, hospital floor. *There is only one direction in which to look.* Gazing out the window upward, toward the heavens, I prayed, "Lord, I don't deserve it, but my heart's desire is to raise my three little boys. I want to see my grandchildren someday. If you will heal me, Lord, I promise to live for you and forever give you the glory." Little did I realize that promise would be challenged time, after time, after time. Compared to what was coming, that experience had only been a prelude.

I WILL FOREVER GIVE HIM THE GLORY

None of you will ever feel
This driving force inside me.
And you may never ever look
At the things that I can see.
But, if you should ever get a glimpse
Of an illness you've had so long
Handle your problems how you may
Then tell me I was wrong.
(Written by: Kittye Sharron)
Author Interpretation:
I'm coming from nowhere to get where I'm going
And the path that I'm taking
Is not even there.
It's something I'm sure of
But there's no way of knowing
If I'll even know when I get there.
(Written by: Kittye Sharron)

CHAPTER 2

The Start of a New Life

*"After the surgery, if I wake up cold
I'll know one of two things: either the
operation was a success or I'm dead!"*

QUOTE BY KITTYE SHARRON (AKA AMY KAYLEEN)

THE NEXT DAY, DURING EXPLORATORY surgery, a rare, baseball size tumor was removed. It was not on either adrenal gland as the doctors had expected; instead the tumor had been attached to my aorta and had been resting on the backbone.

When I woke up in ICU (Intensive Care Unit), I was cold; in fact I was shivering so badly that my teeth were chattering. When the nurse came over to me, I asked her if she was an angel. She had on a white uniform, white rimmed glasses, and her white hair was pulled up neatly. Her stockings and shoes were also white. So, at first glance it looked to me as if there were clouds around her. *I must be in heaven!*

She told me I was being administered strong medication and that the reason I was cold was because I had a high fever. Normally, a patient with a high temperature isn't given a blanket but, when the doctor came by to check on me, he told the nurse to give me anything I wanted. *Imagine that!*

I said, "I haven't been able to use a blanket for so long; may I have one?"

I was given a warm blanket and I slept like a swaddled baby in that bed. I didn't care if it was a hospital bed; it was softer than a bathtub, and it was the first time I had been able to sleep comfortably for a long, long time. Cold water had been my cover for 6 + years, so it was pure joy to feel the softness once again of a real blanket. Even though I had an incision all the way across my abdomen and it hurt to move, I was so thankful the tumor had been found and I was no longer perspiring.

"Lord…, if you're listening, thank you!"

My case was written up in the medical journal in 1974.

Excerpt from my medical records regarding Operative Procedure:
"Pre-operative diagnosis: Pheochromocytoma
Post-operative diagnosis: Left Para ganglion Pheochromocytoma

"To the left of the vertebra, about 3 finger breaths above the vibrication of the aorta to the left of the aorta and overlying the left ureter there arose a large tumor the size of a hard baseball which had a capsule into which ran a tremendously dilated vein with this mass being of a firm nature without showing any evidence of cystic degeneration and without infiltration to the surrounding area. This tumor arose in the position of the left Para ganglionic region between the takeoff of the inferior mesenteric artery and the vibrication of the aorta. The tumor itself had tremendously enlarged veins the size of a pencil and one of such veins directly overlaid the ureter and was because of this, the ureter was injured and transected at the time of removal of the tumor despite the fact the ureter had been previously identified somewhat lateral to this position, prior to this excision."

It went on to say:

"The left adrenal was then approached by an attempt to mobilize the spleen medically together with the tail of the pancreas with an access to the adrenal area could be obtained from the lateral approach. In so doing, a couple of vano veins were inadvertently torn and 1 in the hilum of the spleen finally necessitated the removal of the spleen itself. When it was found that both adrenals were normal, that portion of the abdomen was abandoned and an examination of the organs of Zuckerkandl and the Para ganglionic area re-explored. The tumor was then immediately found without difficulty and vascular supply to the tumor was brought under control and ligated with Polydek suture. When it was discovered that the ureter had been severed, this was then repaired. Patient sustained the procedure without difficulty although at one time, upon the clamping of the last vein of the Pheochromocytoma, pressure drop was anticipated and 3 liters of Ringer's lactate were rushed in the Venus system by the anesthesiologist in very rapid succession. She was discharged to the ICU in good condition."

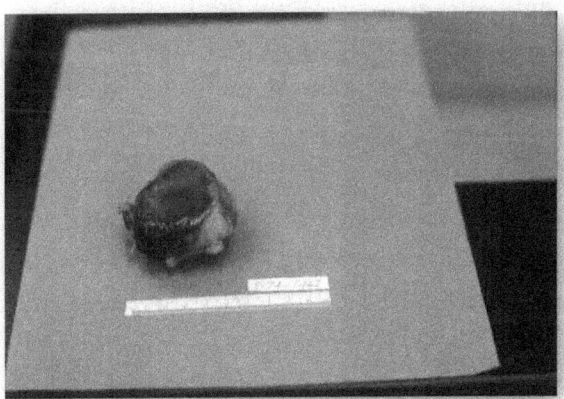

Picture of the Pheochromocytoma tumor which was removed in 1974. It had been attached to the aorta and was resting on the backbone.

To the surprise of the entire surgical team, the tumor was benign. They surmised that it had probably been there my whole life and, during the birth of my first baby, it had begun to grow. Because of the extensive search for the tumor, my spleen, accidentally severed, had to be excised. Once the surgery was over, my blood pressure returned to a normal level, I stopped the profuse perspiring and, after a month long stay in the hospital, on September 1st, 1974, I was discharged. *Mama stayed for a couple of weeks longer to care for the boys until I was able to regain my strength.*

Interestingly, a few years later, I happened to run into that dermatologist who had diagnosed the Pheochromocytoma. I said, "Doctor, do you remember me?" His response, "How could I ever forget someone who slept in a bathtub full of cold water and called me a quack?"

Though that was a very humbling experience, I wish I could tell you I began living for the Lord after that.

Seven and a half years of marriage ended in divorce. Again, I felt embarrassed, lost, and, even though I had been blessed with 3 wonderful little boys, I felt so alone and uneasy. Instead of turning to God, I turned to cigarettes, alcohol, marijuana, men and self. (Years later I would discover, some of those choices could have resulted in my sudden death.) *How God knew to send Jayda Ann into my life at that time is beyond believable. In spite of our wild ways, she was often my protector. There were a few instances, whereby she actually kept me from being harmed and/or harassed.*

I always thought Jayda Ann was so pretty. She, like me, was part Indian. Jayda Ann had high cheek bones, flawless skin, and her long fingernails, which she kept polished red, really showed up on her tanned complexion. She, too, was going through a divorce, had two small children and was just as mixed up as I was. We wore the same hairstyle, both depending on hot rollers to add a little bounce to our long, dark strands. It was always very flattering to me when people would think we were related. Maybe it was because we both liked to dance. Our hip wiggling moves were done on a floor surrounded by flashing squares at a local night spot. Popular dance crazes consisted of The Bump, The Locomotion, The Hustle, The Swing and of course, our favorite, The Twist. *None require learning a lot of complicated steps and have some of the most incredulous moves you've ever seen!*

Along with child support, ADC (Aid to Dependent Children,) and food stamps, I also typed at home in my spare time for one of the psychiatrists in town. That helped pay the bills, but money was tight; going out meant that in order to stretch our meager dollars, Jayda Ann and I would often share the same babysitter. What bad decision one of us didn't think of the other one did. She could talk me out of, and into, almost anything.

Her dog, whom she lovingly named Datch, had puppies and she convinced me to take one home to my kids. *What was I thinking? Puppies have to be fed, house broken, bathed, etc.* Well, I named mine Sassy; the boys loved her.

We had a little circle of friends, about 5 of us who were divorced, all just trying to find our way toward life. It's not that we were bad; we just made bad decisions (*which only makes for great stories!*) So far removed from righteousness, we even laughed at one of our friends who thought her astrological sign was her religious affiliation. When asked which denomination she was, her response was, "Oh, I'm a Capricorn!" *Even though that sounded funny, now it's sad to think we actually found humor in that.*

Jayda Ann didn't drive so I was the designated driver. I had an old clunker of a car that we named "Blue Baby" and many days entertainment was just a drive over to Jayda Ann's house. She had a contagious laugh, which usually had a way of lifting my spirits. A few teen girls enjoyed congregating at her house, too; they thought we had exciting lives. They didn't realize that we actually enjoyed listening to their high school drama. Sometimes we'd wish we could go back in life just to feel a few things twice. *Many things I'd do a lot differently.* We had more in common with them than they realized; all of us were just "little girls" at heart.

The teenagers were always scheming to see what tricks they could play on us, *I think there were many occasions when we were their entertainment.* Once, one of them tossed a full bag of groceries in Jayda Ann's pathway while she was walking backwards. It was a cold, blizzardy day and to avoid the freezing wind in her face, Jayda Ann had turned around when she and the teens were walking to her house from the store. When the back of her feet plowed into that grocery bag, down she went, causing the bag she was carrying to rip; groceries flew everywhere, and most of everything soft was squashed. Mad as she pretended to be, it wasn't long before squeals and laughter were in the air. All but her dozen eggs survived that day; they became raw, yellow snowballs! Her kids ate oatmeal and cinnamon toast for breakfast the rest of that week, even though the slices of bread didn't quite fit right in the toaster!

Since neither of us had much money, what little we could spare usually bought us a pack of cigarettes and a few drops of gas for the car. What was left over was spent for a babysitter, and a round or two at the nightclub. In the mid 70's a pack of cigarettes cost about 45 cents and gas averaged about 57 cents a gallon. *Nowadays, that sounds low; back then it was considered a lot of money to a divorced mother.*

Two women alone in a nightclub filled with strangers can be a dangerous place. *We just want to dance to the music.* We watched each other's back and, when the night was over, always made sure the other was in tow. How she managed to get us kicked out of the bar one night, I never did know, and she could never remember! I could tell you stories which would make a comic laugh *(Jayda Ann would have my head on a platter, because they were mostly about her!) So, I'll just tell you an 'us' story.*

Taking our kids to church was something Jayda Ann and I, together, tried only once. With her son, daughter, and my 3 boys, she and I sheepishly entered the place of worship and sat in a pew near the back of the sanctuary.

The way I remember that dreadful day was that, during prayer, one of our unzipped purses tipped over onto the floor beneath us, spilling out a bunch of change (mostly pennies, several nickels, some thin little dimes, and a few quarters.) (*Plop; clatter, clatter; clink, clink, and clink!*) We immediately bent over and began picking up our precious coins; and if that wasn't bad enough, a pack of cigarettes landed on the floor. While trying to keep our composure we struggled to pick up every last coin (some had rolled under the pew in front of where we sat, *dimes are hard to pick up off a wooden floor!*)

Though out of place and red faced, it was difficult for us and our kids not to burst with laughter. *Shhh…you kids be quiet!* People on each side and in front of our pew were focusing on us instead of praying! We were glad when the service was over, certainly not one of our proudest moments. *Nope, not going back there! Not ever!*

Jayda Ann ended up marrying a very nice guy, moved further north and, except for the exchange of a yearly Christmas card, we just sort of lost touch with one another. She always impressed me with the hand-made, beautiful cards she sent, with her calligraphy resembling fine art.

One cannot go through some of the crazy things we did without remaining forever friends. We were reunited briefly at the funeral of one of the teenagers who babysat our kids, who had died suddenly of an aneurism. After that our lives went in different directions and we saw less and less of each other.

I had dated a few guys, and it always ended badly. The last one was the last straw!

Bill and I met in a bar. He was the bartender, I was the fly! In no way was I looking to meet anyone, since I had just sworn off any kind of relationship and figured I would just drink away my problems. I had no idea I was looking for ways to draw closer to God, but I think that's exactly where I was headed! *I always did take the long way!*

Why Bill was attracted to me, I never could figure out. In spite of where I was that night, I wasn't much of a drinker, never liked the taste and couldn't hold my liquor, so I ordered a straight shot with a coke on the side. After downing the jigger of Southern Comfort with one gulp, and almost falling off the barstool, I began sipping the cola and immediately lit a cigarette. *I just remember the bartender saying, "I'd pay to see that again," and he bought me another drink. Can't show my weakness!* Just to get rid of it, I downed that one, too. *Whew, it's hot in here!*

It was a good thing I was riding with one of my friends, since two drinks was way over my limit. With the exception of having to yell, "Whoa, STOP!" at every corner so I could throw up, I don't even remember the trip home!

I heard later, Bill's brother had been standing on the opposite side of the room and Bill pointed me out to him and said, "You see that girl at the end of the bar? I'm gonna marry her!" His brother said, "You don't want to do that; I hear she's got 3 kids!"

Bill ended up getting my phone number from a friend of mine and called to invite me on a canoe trip. I told him, "no," and further explained to him that I didn't know anything about canoeing and besides, 'I don't like water!' He assured me I could just sit in the canoe, wouldn't have to get wet and it wasn't necessary for me to do anything; just go and he would do all the work! *He is quite the charmer!* Hesitantly, I finally agreed to go.

Still don't know what it was he saw in me, but I know what it was I saw in him, a real 'Daniel Boone' type guy. Strong, tall, soft-spoken, man of few words, handsome, a little rough around the edges but a nice gentle guy…and he did do all the work! While occasionally sipping from a flask of tequila, Bill paddled us comfortably through the winding river without my getting one drop of water on my body during the canoe ride.

Sitting at the front of the canoe, wearing a skimpy bikini, my long hair blowing in the wind, I managed to get bitten on the side of my face by a deer fly, *to which I'm allergic;* my eye was practically swollen shut. Bill acted like he didn't even notice how badly my face looked, *such a sweetheart!*

You know, as long as I was in the boat with him, I was fine. He got us safely to shore but after getting out and realizing I had left my tennis shoes in the canoe, I got back in to retrieve them. *One should never sit on the edge of a canoe, take it from me!* I sat down to put my shoes on and the canoe tipped over with me in it! Bill said all he could see were bubbles rising to the surface of the water! After my 3rd time coming up for air, he, ever so gently, fished me out!

We went nightclubbing a few times after that and to the drive-in movies. Too, there were a few parties which we attended with mutual friends. We took the boys and his daughter to the beach front of Lake Michigan for a few picnics and let the kids all play together while we sat on the blanket and *I talked*. Then, we took a long drive and *I talked* some more, but I don't think either of us had really intended for those dates to be anything serious. You see, prior to our meeting and long before the canoe trip, Bill had already purchased for himself a one way ticket to Hawaii where he was intent on staying. In fact, he flew out just a few weeks after our canoe trip date. I said goodbye with this:

ALOHA, I'LL MISS YOU...
What can I say except, I'll miss you
As you go in search of something new.
Whatever you're seeking I hope you find
If nothing else may it be peace of mind.
We all should find an island
Which we could call our own
And leave all other things behind
So our troubles would be gone.
But the island would eventually sink

As we built our impossible dreams
As with all dreams we don't stay within our means.
Because we want
For bigger and better things
And we keep on building
To see what it brings.
Then...
We search for a different island
And leave the old one behind
Taking with us our peace of mind.
Good luck to you in the "Paradise of the Pacific."
Aloha.

(Written by: Kittye Sharron, AKA Amy Kayleen, in 1976, given to Bill when he left for Hawaii before being in a committed relationship.)

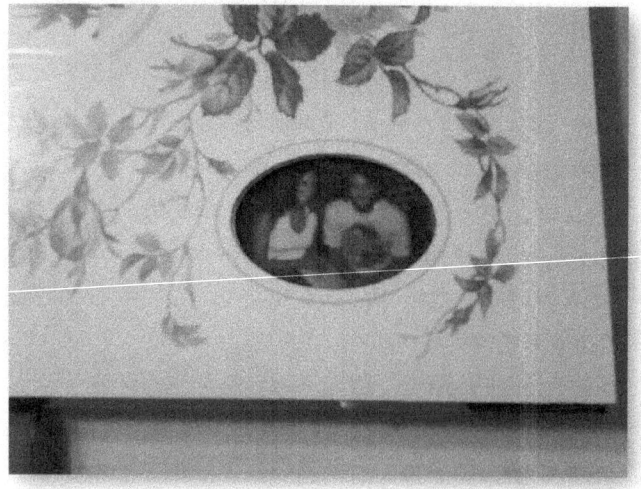

Me (AKA Amy Kayleen) with Bill before he left for Hawaii. (1977)

After he left town, I was sad but I thought of a very good reason why I shouldn't miss him: "He didn't even like to dance!"

I did do some modeling of wedding dresses and make-up; but most of my time was spent taking Criminal Justice courses at the community college in preparation to become a probation officer or maybe a detective; I'd always had an investigative nature. I didn't figure I'd ever hear from Bill again.

That is, of course, until I got that very first letter from him. Then another. We fell in love through those letters and it wasn't long before he was back in Muskegon.

His loving proposal will forever resonate in my heart: "Well, we might as well get hitched!" *(Even though he is of Michigan descent, Bill's persona reminds me of John Wayne's in the movie, The Quiet Man.)*

Doesn't he know what he's getting himself into? (3 kids, stubborn, outspoken woman!)

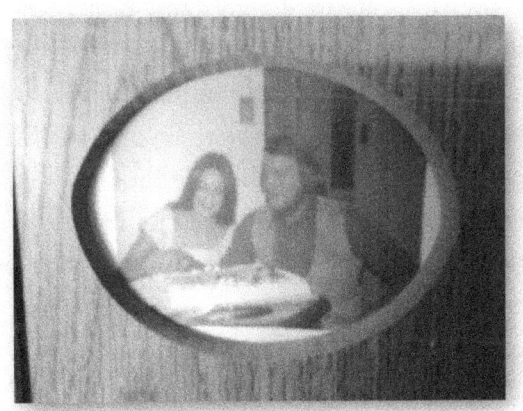

Wedding Day Cake, December 21, 1977.
Bill & me (AKA Amy Kayleen)

We were married by the Justice of the Peace at the courthouse on December 21st, 1977. It was a cold, blustery, teeth-chattering Wednesday afternoon; I wore a plain off-white dress, which I had borrowed from a friend. Bill looked quite dapper; beige, corduroy pants, matching vest over a long-sleeved dark brown shirt... *Hard to believe, at the time, Bill's light brown hair was almost as long as mine!* After the ceremony, we had a small reception at our motel room. We couldn't afford much; *someday we'll go on a honeymoon*; several of our friends stopped by with whom we partied into the night; that is, until Bill announced, "Party's over!" and everybody left. *My man of few words!*

Not long after our wedding we gained custody of Bill's ten year old daughter. We decided right then and there, what was his and mine would become 'ours.' That's how I got my beautiful girl...*now my daughter* who, with dark brown hair and big brown eyes, actually had many of my features.

Having already discovered our common ground.....party, party, party, that's what Bill and I did every other weekend when our kids would be at their other parent's house. We wallowed in that muddy lifestyle for a few years.

It was Bill's mother who spoke to us about the Lord, and suggested we take a good look at the way were living. Bill and I began to talk about it and started praying together. We wanted to do right and, just when we thought we had it licked, one of our old friends would come over and we would fall right back into temptation.

Toward the end of 1981, we made an effort to start new lives. *This was a trial run of my newly found trust for the Lord.*

At that time, the economy looked bleak and many establishments had gone out of business; rumor had it ours would be next. Therefore, neither of us felt secure in our positions. Bill had previously stopped being a bartender and had taken a factory job as a spray painter. I had quit college by then and worked at the phone company, first in Central Files, then promoted to the Customer Service department as a secretary.

In addition to layoff threats, Bill's job had horrible effects on his lungs. Having already received a serious injury to his nose a few months prior, he really wanted to get out of that place.

I, on the other hand, loved my job but the merging of the phone company in Indiana with the one in Muskegon, where I worked, had already taken place. Jobs were being eliminated and my position felt less than stable.

Given the facts, taking into consideration we had four hungry little mouths to feed and a poodle/mix dog, we began discussing what would be in our best interests and where we might like to relocate. Our decision: Florida, here we come!

Our mothers and Mama took care of the kids and Sassy and, while in an effort to scope out the Florida job market, Bill and I left for a deferred honeymoon/vacation. On a cold, snowy day, driving our old '69 red and white Fleetwood Cadillac (that we had bought used) we headed toward Ft.

Lauderdale to visit Bill's grandmother who spent her winters there. In addition to her home in Muskegon, she owned a spacious, 2-bedroom condo at the gated River Reach Condominiums situated on the intercostal waterway. It was a free place to stay and, on our budget, free was always good.

Bill wanted to take a detour, to stop in Naples and pay a visit to an ex-brother-in-law. That's where it started. Our car broke down! We were stranded in Naples, Florida, free room at the ex's, and we loved every minute of it. It became clear that's where we wanted to live.

After a few days in the garage our car was back running and we made our way across Alligator Alley to spend the remainder of our vacation at Bill's grandmother's condominium.

It was a real treat. Pure delight was ours as we sun bathed while lounging by the pool, sweated in the sauna, then cooled ourselves in the water while floating on a raft. After a few hours, we would shower in the bath house, and stroll back to Nan's. She had a little wooden rack out on her patio where we hung our wet bathing suits to dry. There we smooched on the swing *(dizzy in love!)*. Into late afternoon, we enjoyed our 'honeymoon' while breathing in the fragrances of warm salty air mixed with the sweet scents drifting from the Night Blooming Jasmine hedges that lined the walkway along the water's edge. After steaks on the grill, munching raw vegetables and sipping freshly squeezed lemonade, we'd wave to the passengers that were on the big tour boat called the River Queen, which floated by every evening. That was Bill's signal to me it was time for bed. *Do not disturb!*

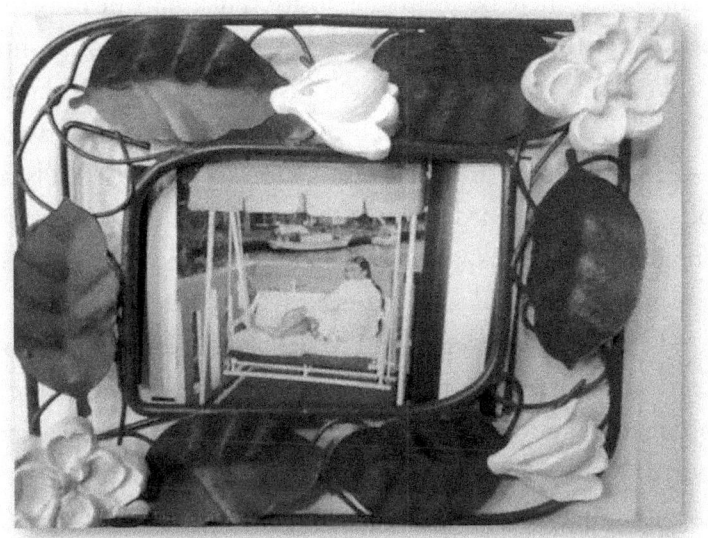

Kittye Sharron (AKA Amy Kayleen) sitting on the swing in Ft. Lauderdale.

Nan was a gracious hostess and seemed to have an inside scoop as to what honeymooning was all about. Not only did she make herself scarce in the evenings, she let us sleep in as long as we wanted to in the mornings. The aromas of coffee brewing and her wonderful cottage cheese waffles with warmed syrup awakened us each morning. All too soon our vacation was over and it became time to do the leg work toward our ambition.

As we had previously decided, Bill would go first. We returned home, he put in his notice at the factory, and two weeks later boarded a plane and headed back to the sunshine state. Once there he secured a position just outside of Naples at a water filtration plant. Our goal was to move our family to Florida. We took steps to do just that, but not without a few obstacles, some of which involved court cases and convincing the judge to grant permission to move the kids out of state; a huge hurdle. After that, in order to comply with the divorce decrees, arrangements had to be made with our ex-spouses to spend summer months with the kids.

I stayed in Muskegon and continued to work at the phone company during the day and afterwards worked at home in order to get the house ready to put on the market. I began burning the candle at both ends… painting walls, preparing for a garage sale, and packing up our belongings, not to mention all the meal preparation and basic care of four adolescents, and a dog, plus maintaining the yard. (*Kids, get your homework done! It's bath time! Bedtime! Grocery shopping! Wash the dishes, then the dog! There's laundry to be done, grass needs mowing, etc.*)

It was during that same time, our daughter called me at work one day to tell me that Sassy was giving birth to puppies. That was definitely an unplanned event, having to find homes for, but first weaning, 4 puppies.

Coworkers and friends were laughing, pointing out that due to the poor economy nobody would buy our house. My response, "I guess the Lord will buy it!" *"You want a free puppy?"*

I worked so hard that I must have lowered my immunity (*that's right, I don't have a spleen!*) After using a tampon I ended up in the hospital for a month with Toxic Shock Syndrome. Once I was discharged, I thought I was out of the woods, went to the dentist for a routine cleaning and had a relapse that resulted in Bacterial Endocarditis and another week in the hospital! (*Enough of this being sick nonsense; I want to get to Florida!*)

In May, 1981, our house sold…it was the Lord's doing! (That became my reason for everything.) *Do I really trust Him?* Testing had only just begun!

We said our goodbyes to family, friends and neighbors. Our furniture had been packed into a moving truck and was headed for a storage unit in Naples. Sadly, we gave our little Sassy to a very nice couple who lived on a farm. Our kids would be staying with their other parent for two months, at which time they would then fly to our new location. Bill had flown home to get me so that we could drive our car to Florida. He was off work since he had accidentally suffered a cut on his hand and was put on temporary disability.

It seemed as though all we had left to do before getting in our car was to wait for the service technician to come and disconnect our telephone. While waiting for that to occur, the phone rang; it was Bill's boss in Florida. He was calling to say that Bill was being dismissed because of leaving the state while on disability; no longer did he have a job!

I lost it! I ran out the back door and crumbled to the ground. Bill followed me. Crying and desperate for an answer, I asked him, "What are we going to do now? Our house is sold, our furniture is on its way to Florida and your job is gone. Where is the Lord now?"

Bill, in all his wisdom said, "We'll be okay, we need to just trust Him." Then he prayed.

That was a new way of life for me. I didn't know how to trust and I surely wasn't very good at that praying thing! We quickly realized we must follow our plans, and all our belongings, so we picked ourselves up, piled into our old car, and off we went, Florida or bust!

The trip was filled with lots of communication, anywhere from discussions regarding the kids, to wondering how many snowflakes it takes to make an inch of snow. We listened and sang along to the top songs on the radio (i.e. "Endless Love" by Diana Ross and Lionel Ritchie; "Just like Starting Over" by John Lennon; "Step-by-Step" and "I Love a Rainy Night", by Eddie Rabbit.)

Oh yes, and that trip was filled with enjoyable romantic kisses on the neck, and a few laughs along the way. Whenever a lull, I often put my head back on the headrest, or practiced the 'Cadillac lean' and as Bill drove I'd occasionally drift off to sleep. Once I woke up suddenly and screamed for I thought for sure there was something frightening alongside the road.

"IT'S A BEAR!" (It was a cow.) *Bill has never let me forget that one and, to this day, it's one of his favorite stories; he's easily humored!*

I had made a plan to quit smoking as soon as we crossed the Florida border. Sure enough, as soon as we saw the sign "Welcome to Florida, The Sunshine State," what few cigarettes that were left in the pack went out the window. As addictions go, of course, I was tempted to buy another pack, but my desire to quit was greater and I decided to replace the habit with something that wouldn't be bad for my health.

It was then I started keeping an ink pen in my pocket and whenever the urge to light up presented itself, I took out my pen and held onto it as if it were a cigarette. I had always heard there was power in the name, Jesus, so I just started whispering "Jesus." The longer I refrained from smoking the less my desire. (*There is more about what I call, "My Red Pen Ministry," in a later chapter toward the back of this book.*)

We estimated a down payment of $1,000 would be required to rent a house, so with some of the money we got from the sale of our home in Michigan we put that amount, plus what we thought first, last and security would be, in the bank not to be touched until we found jobs. The home in Michigan had been sold on a land contract so a house payment from the buyers would be forthcoming every month, which offered us a little security. But until the kids were to arrive two months later, we rented a cheap, little efficiency apartment which was on the outskirts of Naples. What money we had on hand bought us groceries and gas; we knew that would have to last us until we could begin bringing in paychecks.

I'm sure you've heard the nursery rhyme of Old Mother Hubbard who went to her cupboard…we had the same thing going for us. Every day we were faced with the possibility that we were doomed. We were living on love, and we clung to each other and together practiced praying. Just when we were, literally, down to only carrots in the bottom of the refrigerator, God sent us an unlikely friend - an overweight retired man who had a bad body odor which he could not help, and a face full of scraggly whiskers, which looked so untidy. His name, Hal. *"…some have entertained angels without knowing it."(Hebrews 13:2b)*

Hal was a friend of Bill's ex brother-in-law and in spite of his appearance he was the nicest person. He began coming over daily. Using his car and his gas he would take us job hunting; afterward we would go to his house for a few hours. Invariably, his sweet wife, Reba, would have a most delicious meal waiting when we arrived.

Together, Hal and Reba had no kids but did have a beagle named Rusty who was allowed to sit on a chair next to the table and eat off a plate that was placed there for him. *One lucky dog!*

It pleased us so much the day Reba saved for us the drippings from a beef brisket and gave us flour to take back to our little efficiency apartment. It made for a delicious breakfast gravy the next day; it's at times like that when one learns how to offer up a prayer of thanksgiving. What we would have done without Hal and Reba, I do not know, but I'm certain God knew we needed them.

In perfect time we each landed a job, got on our feet and became very busy. Bill was hired at a life care facility and worked his way up to maintenance foreman. I had taken a job as a private secretary but would eventually be offered a position as Executive Housekeeper at the same place Bill worked. *What's an Executive Housekeeper? (The Executive Housekeeper directs and controls all housekeeping operations and the staff of the housekeeping department. He/she has to coordinate between housekeeping crews in order to inspect assigned areas and to ensure standards.)* I was told it required someone with good organizational skills. *Who me?* I could hardly turn it down since, just to start, the pay was almost twice as much as I could expect in my clerical position.

The summer was over; the kids arrived just a few days after we rented our first 4 bedroom house in a suburb of Naples, called Golden Gate. We lived there for a year and after that were able to rent a house on the other side of Golden Gate Parkway which was a little bigger and much nicer. There was a canal in the back where an occasional wildlife critter would be observed. When not in school, the kids enjoyed trying to catch whatever would be out there.

One year a "No Name" storm hit; it rained so much that the canal was up to our back door and the driveway had so much flooding that the floorboard of our car had standing water. Neighbors were using boats to get to the main road. The kids were happy that the schools closed for a week and they got to swim in the streets, that is until a snake was the doing the same!

Bill had been raised to attend church, I couldn't claim one. Wanting so badly to worship the Lord, I told my husband I would follow his lead. We began going to a church but I felt like I didn't belong. The many rituals seemed very strange to me. I didn't know when to stand up or sit down, or whether to turn around or do a flip! *God will you help me?*

Every Sunday, after the service, I had my favorite window in our bedroom where I would stand and pray. Looking out toward the canal, I told the Lord that I was sorry I didn't understand and I asked Him to either change my heart or change the circumstances.

For about a year, I prayed that same prayer, and God had been listening. After church one Sunday, Bill said that he was not being fully fed spiritually. He suggested we try going to the one in which our friends attended. The following week, that is exactly what we did.

I heard something that sounded strangely familiar. It was a message I had heard as an adolescent, the gospel. I learned that I was not defined by my failure nor my past, and that Jesus must be the anchor of my heart.

It was there I realized I was a sinner and there was nothing I could do to save myself, but that Jesus had died for my sins. Though undeserving, I had been given everything: eternal life given by God's grace for people like me. Despite who I was, what had happened to me when I was a child, or things I had done...*doesn't matter, Jesus loves me, the sinner!*

Once again, I prayed and asked the Lord to forgive me. I invited Him into my heart. Bill did the same and we went forward that day, September 25th, 1983, made a public profession of faith, and got baptized that very night.

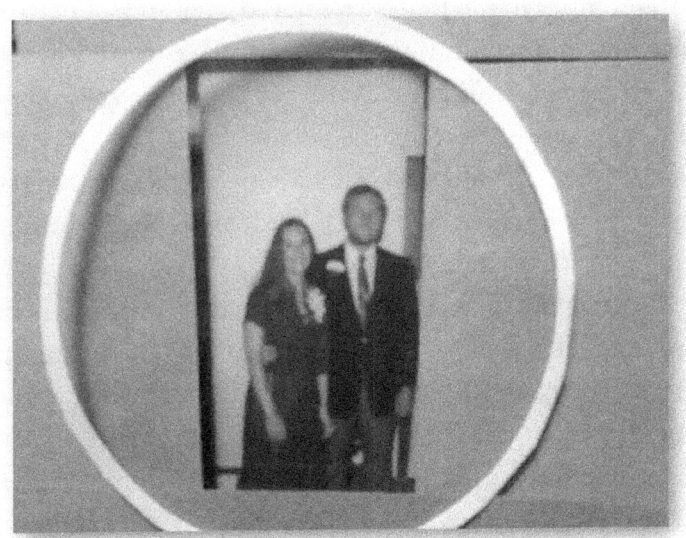

Kittye Sharron, (AKA Amy Kayleen), and Bill ~ Vow Renewal Ceremony, December 21, 1983

It was at that same church, three months later on a Wednesday afternoon, December 21st, 1983, our 6th wedding anniversary, we rededicated our marriage vows in the presence of God.

Bill surprised me with a lovely corsage, containing white roses and Lily of the Valley, which he gently pinned on the bodice of the burgundy dress I wore. He was all decked out in a dark blue suit with a matching tie and a pink shirt. His hair by then had been cut short and it was neatly combed. *A far cry from our first ceremony!* All 4 of our children were present, along with the minister, his wife, and our new church family. After our Christian ceremony, to celebrate our solemn promises to the Lord, we enjoyed cake and ice cream in the fellowship hall until it was time for Wednesday evening church to begin. When we returned home, before going to bed, we played the card game Uno with our kids.

We went faithfully to church every Sunday morning, every Sunday evening, and every Wednesday night for many years. Sin still found us!

When not working, I busied myself in the local poetry club, ran for and was elected Secretary. I had written poetry for years and it was a way for me to grow in the art. The definition of poetry being: words written in a way to please the ear; and the philosophy behind it: anyone can be a poet…'take a word, write a line, and have it end in a rhyme'. Writing and reciting my poetry put me on center stage at area events. One of my fondest memories was when two of my sons escorted me off stage after a performance, one on each side of me. I felt so honored.

There was nothing wrong with what I was doing, except I got too busy doing it. In addition, I was involved in church things, career things, focusing on the yard, fashion, and raising 4 teenagers. I became preoccupied with the house, the dog, the cat (***and we didn't even have a cat or a dog at that time; they belonged to the neighbor!***) Anything and everything became something of a hectic routine.

You see, I had my priorities mixed up! It wasn't long before Bible reading had begun to taper off. I wasn't spending time with God or meditating on His Word. Old ways of thinking threatened me, but I didn't want to wander away from the gospel again.

That did not last long; my faith in Jesus Christ sustained me. He convicted me! I had felt lost when I fell out of fellowship with Him and didn't know how to get it back. Help in recovering from that came in the form of a Christian overcomers support group. I learned new skills by attending weekly meetings and began to apply those to my life. Again, I confessed, asked the Lord to forgive me, and I repented of my wrongdoings. I began to understand that Christ was sent as a substitute for my sins. That's why we need a Savior. He died in my place (*and yours.*) I realized that I needed to spend the rest of my life learning about Him and what He did for me. He died so that I may live. There was nothing I could do to change my past, but Jesus had changed my future.

The awful thing that happened to me as a child of 8 was just that; it was awful being victimized by a pedophile. I had been defiled, *but it doesn't define me. That doesn't make me who I am or ever was. It's what I do with Jesus that matters.* He got me through it. When I gave that burden to the Lord, the weight of the world seemed lifted from my shoulders. *(Chapter 9 explains how that was accomplished.)* There is no room for shame, bitterness and anger in the gospel, and no need to run away from God. *I'm a child of the King! Jesus is God and He resides in my heart. He is Immanuel (which means God with us.) I have joy and I live in His strength.*

In fact, the Lord kept me alive. His supernatural strength pulled me out of many frightening and sinful situations. As a result, I have experienced joy, shock, relief and gratitude, just to name a few. It is through people that God accomplishes much. "From everyone who has been given much, much will be required." (Luke 12:48). *I think, when a person has been through much, they should give God the glory and write a book, or two, or three!*

CHAPTER 3

How Poor was Poor?

BURDETTE, ARKANSAS S ~ BEGINNING 35 YEARS EARLIER (1948)

THE TRUTH IS, LIFE IS full of challenges and when I think back to how far the Lord has brought me, it brings me to my knees. I began to see how He had me in the palm of His hand all along. May I never forget my humble beginnings!

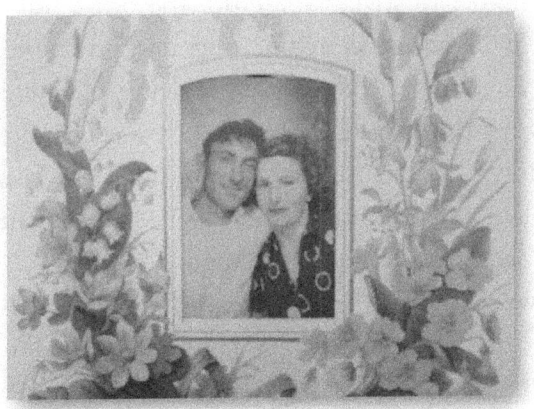

My father and mother were married on January 19, 1947 in Luxora, Arkansas.

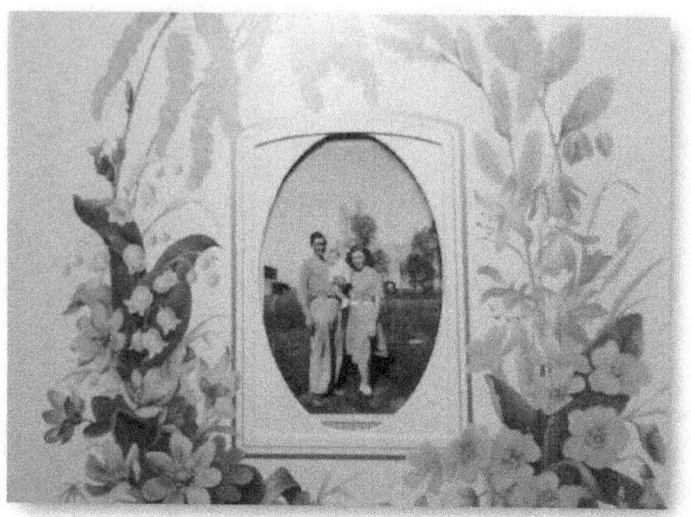

Pictured is my father, holding me (AKA Amy Kayleen), and my mother (AKA Peggy Marie) in 1948.

Reminiscing, I often looked back to the early days of how mine began…May 1st, 1948, the day I was born, my mother lovingly had shared her memories with me.

It was Saturday, 6:00 a.m. She felt a nice warm breeze blowing gently through the open screened windows of the old country farmhouse. She could smell the scent of her freshly laundered curtains and enjoyed the softness of the feather bed in which she was lying.

However, things were not so calm under the covers, since inside her something was about to break…her water! Until contractions started, she thought she had wet the bed.

A race to get from the country to the city of Blytheville in his old, black Ford became my dad's wake up call. Wall's Hospital was approximately nine miles away - *no expressway*.

Born a few hours later, I became my daddy's little girl. Apparently, I was born with lots of dark hair that matched his, and my big eyes were almost black. Mother said I was perfect! She claimed my face was perfectly shaped and pretty (*don't all mothers say that?*).

Mother also said when they got me home, I cried a lot, like I was in pain. The doctor diagnosed me with colic. It became quite a ritual, *I suppose very stressful,* both of them trying to calm a crying baby, but I was the apple of both sets of eyes and I loved both of them.

My parents were poor. They picked cotton and would haul me around on the back of a cotton sack. (*To this day, I love the smell of freshly picked cotton.*) We lived on a partially graveled/dirt road on the outskirts of Blytheville in a little town called Burdette. We even had a big male dog by the name of Jody. When we were not in the fields of cotton and it was time for my nap, Mother would lay me in my bassinette on the screened in porch as she went about her inside chores.

Jody became my dependable body guard. Once, a door-to-door saleswoman who was trying to sell vanilla flavoring, made an effort to come onto the porch of our house while I slept. Jody saw to it that it wouldn't be so easy and would not allow her anywhere near the porch. He barked, howled and showed her his teeth. Everything became fine once Mother came to the door, called Jody's name, and said, "Hush."

Jody didn't always present himself as a threat and was well known to the salesmen who would bring their goods to the little store at the end of our road. When Jody would wander down there, the salesmen would always give him bubble gum, which he chewed until the sweetness was gone.

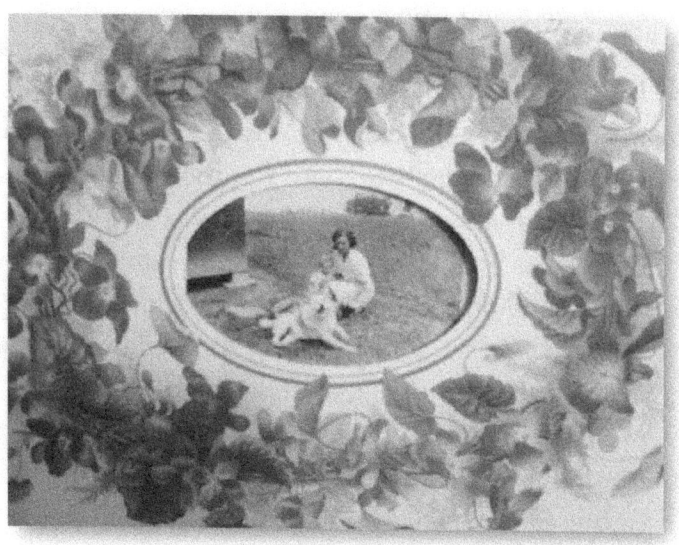

Dog Jody, Mama and, baby me (AKA Amy Kayleen.)

Mama and Nanny were my maternal grandparents *(just a note here: everyone in our family referred to my grandmother as 'Mama.' Before I was born my grandfather wanted to be called, 'Granddaddy'; however, when I started talking it came out, 'Nanny,' and that's who he was from then on! In memory of him, I carry on that tradition today; my grandchildren call me Nanny.)* Prior to moving to Michigan, they lived across the railroad tracks from the country store. Nanny told a lot of funny stories about Jody; one in particular was when he offered to show an elderly black man that Jody could smile. The old man quickly spoke up and said, "Oh that's alright; I never did like a dog laughing at me."

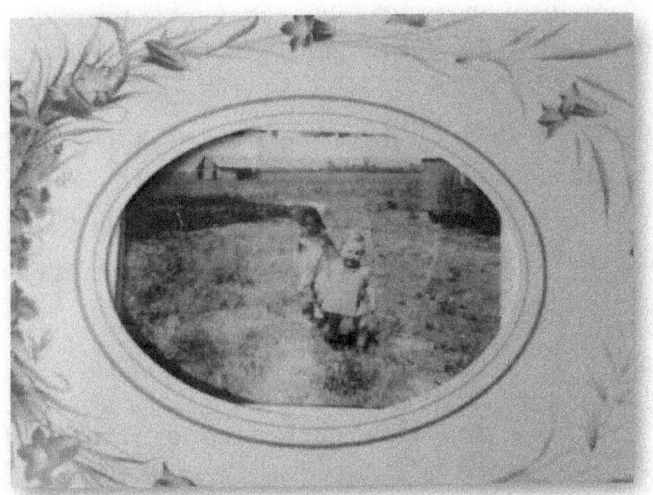

Toddlers: AKA Amy Kayleen wearing a bonnet. In front, AKA Robyn Louise. (Our back yard in Burdette, Arkansas.)

I had been the first grandchild on my mother's side of the family; my little sister, Robyn Louise, came along 22 months later. (Mother said she was pretty, too.)

When the cotton was out of season my parents and grandparents would pack up what few belongings our car would hold, (the rest of which, along with Jody, was given away to one of the other cotton pickers), and we headed north for Michigan where they would pick fruit. One year we lived in a tent. (*To this day, those are cherished memories and probably the reason I love camping.*)

The cherry orchard became Robyn's and my playground. The scraping of tree limbs as they hit the side of the car when we drove down the orchard's trail became one of my favorite sounds. About midday we would eat while sitting on one of Mother's freshly laundered sheets (*washed by hand using a scrub board*), which she would spread on the ground under the cool shade of a cherry tree. Lunch usually consisted of canned Vienna sausages or sardines, cheese, peanut butter and crackers or plain bologna between two slices of white loaf bread.

We slept on a quilt pallet and always went to bed clean. In the evening, after a long, hard day, and prior to going to bed, Mother would "scrub" our feet trying to get the dirt off our olive colored skin only to discover, underneath the dirt, were tan lines that wouldn't wash off. That didn't keep her from trying, even during our complaints, ("Ow, ow, ow!") She had a fair complexion and didn't realize we took after our dad (*in more ways than one, we would eventually discover.) It was not at all unusual for my sister to have a bandage on her head. She managed to trip and fall on numerous occasions, and she was always spilling her milk. Years later, eye glasses made a huge difference.*

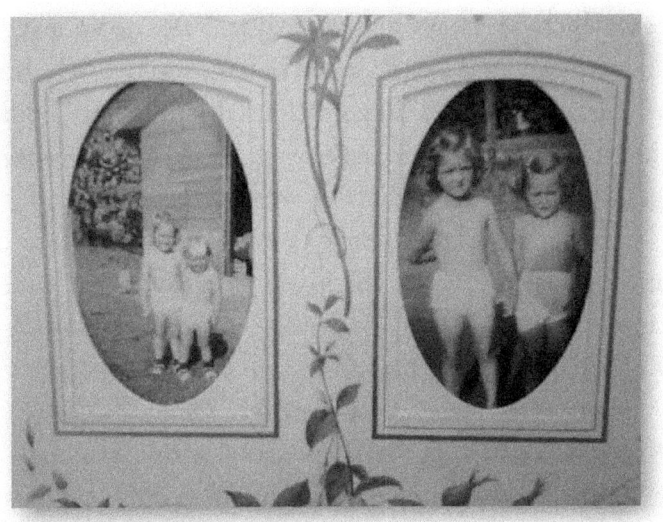

Picture above: In Michigan, from one year to the next. After our baths, left to right: AKA Amy Kayleen and AKA Robyn Louise. 1951 & 1952.

The following year my parents got indoor jobs while in Michigan, and we moved up in the world, living in a one-room house next to the canning factory where they worked. It didn't have running water inside, but outside there was a pump which was handy for drinking and taking pan baths. We had electricity inside our little dwelling, which allowed an electric skillet to be used for cooking. Mother ingeniously designed Robyn's and my bed by putting two overstuffed, upholstered chairs together.

When payday came for Mother and Dad, we would go to a little hole-in-the wall restaurant and my dad would order a hot beef sandwich with mashed potatoes and brown gravy, which he always shared with me. Oh, how I loved my dad; from the food he ate, to his radiant smile, bright brown eyes, bulging muscles, huge calloused hands, the jubilance in his voice, his gait; *I think I even loved the ground he walked on and, would forever chase the footprints he left behind.*

Afterward, we got to enjoy a strawberry ice cream cone from the Dairy Castle, which was situated on the street in front of our little abode. *(Strawberry remains my favorite flavor of ice cream; and I never look at a hot beef sandwich that I don't think of my dad; to this day I love brown gravy.)*

In spite of our less than luxurious temporary one room home, those were happy days for me. Both my parents were working together, I was content, and we were a family of four.

My sweet mother worked alongside my father daily and didn't stop when we got home. Cooking, cleaning, and bathing us every night… her hands were chafed from using a washboard to keep our clothing clean…*I don't know how she did it. She wanted better for us than what she had growing up. My maternal grandfather was an alcoholic and she always vowed she would never tolerate that.*

One thing I remember about my dad was how badly he would perspire. I always thought it was because he worked so hard. It wasn't until later in life I would discover the real reason and how much he and I truly had in common.

After the growing season was over for cherries, peaches, pears, beans, cucumbers, tomatoes and apples in Michigan, we would head back south to Arkansas in the fall for my parents to once again pick more cotton. That was the year Mama and Nanny stayed in Michigan to live permanently. Oh, how we missed them.

Soon after we were back in Arkansas, my dad got a job driving a truck for a local meat distributor, but that was short lived. Alcohol soon began controlling his every action, so much so that he chose it over his wife and daughters. Therefore, our circumstances changed drastically.

The white house in which we lived was on Clarke Street, and we could see the railroad tracks from our front yard. Mother had a job as a waitress at a restaurant within walking distance. It was on that street where I learned to ride a bike and on that same street life as I had always known it, would be no more.

One dark night, my father, who was in a drunken stupor, became abusive toward my mother; it hadn't been the first time. The little girl in me wondered, "What's happening to my daddy? This is so unlike him." After he fell asleep, my mother, my sister and I each put all our earthly treasures in a paper bag and we walked away in the middle of the night. We ended up at the home of a sweet, elderly woman who my mother knew. She gave us shelter, a bed in which to sleep and, to me (after wiping away my tears) she gave a bed doll. I named her Nancy. In fact, after that I named every doll I ever got Nancy. (*Go figure, to this very day, I still have every one of them in my doll cabinet in the living room of my house!*

The old bed doll is Nancy with a broken leg; Nancy Blue, of course, has blue hair and wears a blue dress; Nancy after-the-wedding doll has on a red velvet 2-piece suit; and Nancy walking doll actually walks!)

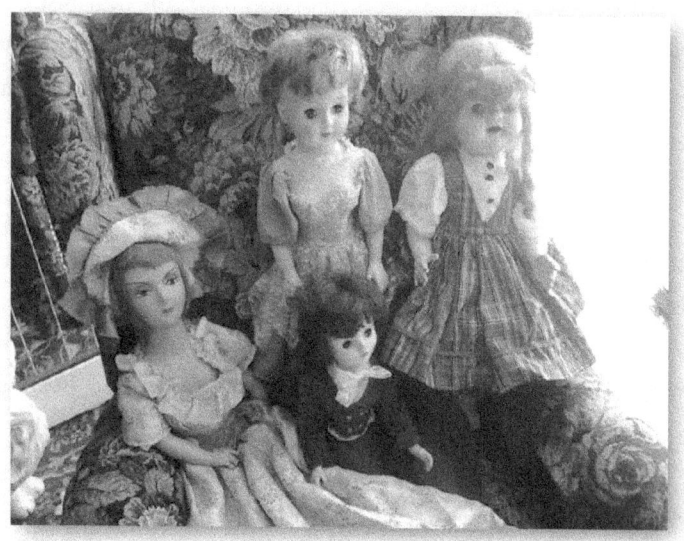

My "Nancy" dolls.

My granddaughters enjoy them when they come. In fact, once when they came to visit, one of them brought me a new doll. I said, "I am going to name her . . . Nancy!" To which she responded, "Nanny, you can't name all your dolls Nancy!"

My parent's divorce became final after they had been separated for two years, and my dad got the car. Mother, Robyn and I moved into a small duplex apartment. It was hard for my mother having to walk to work, walk while at work, and walk back home from work; she was on her feet all day, just to make ends meet; but she managed to provide for my sister and me on her slim salary and tips. We never went to bed hungry; Mother made sure of that. At the time, she had one waitress uniform and one apron, which she washed by hand and starched (liquid starch; no spray starch back then,) every night; she ironed them before going to work every morning. Too, she kept her white shoes polished and regularly washed the shoe strings.

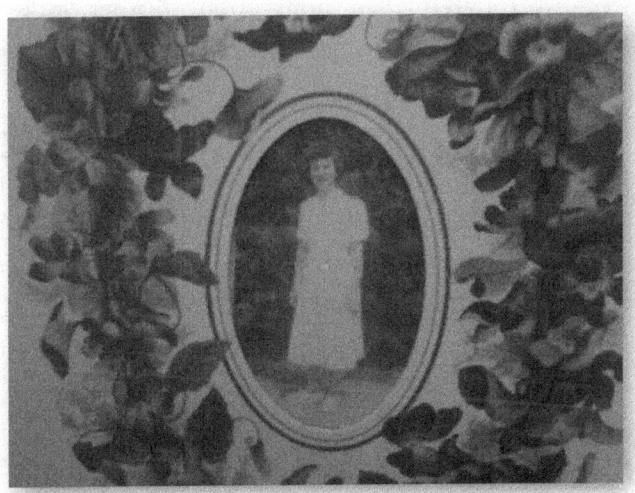

Mother (AKA Peggy Marie) in her neatly pressed waitress uniform and polished white shoes.

Even though I was just a little girl, I sensed she could use help, but mine wasn't always appreciated. We had an old wringer washer at that time. I had watched Mother use it and was just sure I could handle the wash. Mother couldn't afford a babysitter to come in, but the lady next door kept an eye on us and was there if we needed anything. While Mother was at work one day, I proceeded to do the laundry. *"I'll surprise Mother!" Oh, she was surprised alright!* Everything was fine until time to let the water drain out. When I pulled the plug, water went everywhere; I flooded the entire duplex, water even seeped into the apartment next door. *What a mess!* Needless to say, that was not a good day, but we got through it, even though poor Mother worked late into the night cleaning up my mess.

There were times that the meat on the table was just fried bologna, but it was meat and we were thankful for it and the flour gravy that my mother made to go with it. ("Thank you, Lord, for our fried bologna, gravy and bread," was the way in which one of our prayers began before our meal. Robyn pronounced it: 'dray' bee'.) We didn't always have packaged loaf bread, but that was okay with Robyn and me; buttermilk biscuits or cornbread were just fine (*and still are!*)

I learned to cook, a little, when I was just 9 years old. Since Mother's job required her to leave early for work, I had to fix breakfast for my sister and me before school. Fried eggs took me a while to master and I ruined many, which had to be thrown away because Robyn wouldn't eat them if I broke the yolk. So I came up with a plan. I had her sit in the living room while I prepared them. Afterward, I would put them on the plate and cut them up before I called her into the kitchen to eat. She never knew the difference and it kept me from wasting eggs.

For supper, a pot of black-eyed peas, seasoned with a strip of bacon if we had it, was put on the stove for many of our meals. Turnip greens on the side was always a hit with me. (Robyn was easily fooled. She thought she only liked mustard greens, but she really didn't know the difference, so that became Mother's and my secret.) The cornbread we had with it, we'd make sure to leave some to crumble afterward into our glass of milk. Many times that was our dessert; other times we had sweet, yummy butter rolls, banana pudding or, my favorite, Mother's blackberry cobbler. Southern fried chicken on Sunday was something we always looked forward to, that is, if Mother made enough money in restaurant tips that week. If not, she always made something which we liked, at least filled our bellies even if it was flour gravy over biscuits and scrambled eggs. *She was, still is, a great cook! (So is my sister!)*

If we went anywhere, we had to walk. Some of my fondest memories include the three of us, after Mother got off work, going to the wrestling matches which were held a short distance from where we lived. I always felt sorry for the underdog; once I went up to a "mean wrestler" by the name of Bernard the Brute and asked him for an autograph. I didn't realize then, it was all for show, but he threw my autograph book on the ground and stomped on it! The crowd laughed;

I was so embarrassed. "How dare you!" I put my hands on my hips, picked up my book and showed him I could stomp away too. *I really needed that autograph for my collection. I never liked him again after that!*

Razorback Restaurant was the name of the place where Mother worked as a waitress. There was a juke box inside and when the 45 rpm records were changed out, she got permission to have the ones they were throwing away, which she brought home. Robyn and I entertained ourselves by playing them over and over again on our little hand-me-down record player. Back in the day, some of our favorites were, Jim Reeves singing, "Roly Poly" and "Have I Told You Lately That I Love You", also Hank Snow singing, "Make the World Go Away"; and Ernest Tubb sang my very favorite, "Soldier's Last Letter"; *the lyrics to which I vividly recall to this day.*

We resided in that small two bedroom apartment for several years before finally relocating to Michigan, but during those years in Blytheville, corndogs at the fairgrounds were considered one of our favorite treats and we could have one ride on the Ferris wheel, which was enough because that was all Mother could afford. Too, that was all my queasy stomach would allow; I upchucked in front of the concession stand once, so after that I didn't care too much for carnival rides. (I always got car sick, too.) It was fun just to walk around and see all the sights.

Regardless of how bad the tips were for her, Mother always made sure Robyn and I had new dresses and hats every Easter for us to wear, not to church because we didn't have one, but when strolling on the sidewalk in front of the "closed for Sunday" storefronts, where we'd go window-shopping. Mother was so proud of my sister and me and would save up money to have a picture made of the three of us. (That was long before the days of digital technology; it wasn't cheap.)

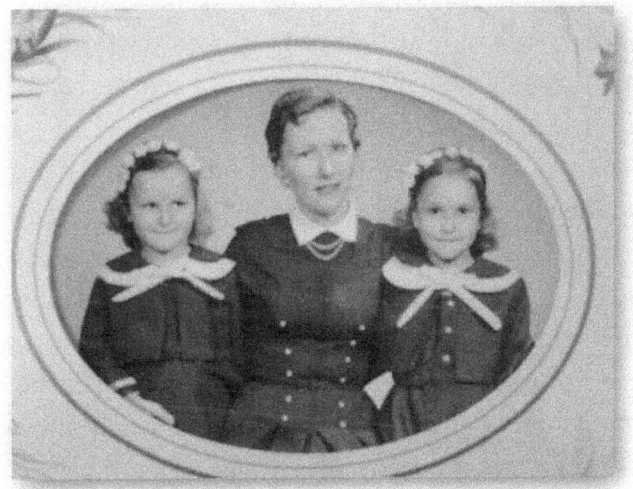

1956, (left to right: AKA Robyn Louise (6), AKA Peggy Marie (27) and me, AKA Amy Kayleen (8).

We always got a new dress on our birthdays, and every Christmas morning Robyn and I each had a new doll under the tree. *(When my mother was growing up, she and my uncles were lucky if they got an orange for Christmas, so she always wanted us to have a better life. To this day, her generosity shows. Though now retired, she still works; crocheting and giving gifts to practically everyone she meets, especially at Christmas.)* We loved skipping on the sidewalks all the way to and from town on holidays. When we boarded the Greyhound Bus for our move from Arkansas to Michigan, I remember peering out the window of the bus and it seemed as though I was saying goodbye to old friends as the sights of those stores and familiar sidewalks got further and further away from my view.

Our first home in Muskegon, was a cement block house on Myrtle Street near a place called Jackson Hill (not the best part of town, and it became quickly apparent to me they didn't like southerners.) *Getting beat up after school a few times because of my accent taught this little girl from Arkansas to put aside her drawl and talk like a Yankee!* Surprisingly, my teacher told me it wasn't necessary to say, "Yes ma'am" whenever she would address me. Luckily for me, one of the older, stronger and wiser classmates took me under her wing and saw to it I got home safely. She was a black girl by the name of Shirley and she made me feel important; taught me valuable lessons which were not stressed where I had come from. Things like: crayons come in different colors as do eyes, hair and skin; never use the "n" word!

My mother met and married my stepfather. It was so nice to finally, once again, have two 'parents' *with a car.* He didn't have any children of his own, but he treated Robyn and me like we were his biological daughters, and we were soon calling him 'Dad'. His and Mother's combined incomes allowed us the opportunity to move to the suburbs. Our house was situated in an attractive neighborhood in Norton Shores – a modest, newly built, three bedroom home, with a full basement.

The basement was where Robyn and I would help Mother can jars of tomatoes and vegetable soup. That is, of course, after we finished shelling butter beans, peas and, snapping green beans. It was also the first and only place my sister ever did anything wrong.

The washer and dryer were down in the basement and Mother would start a wash load of clothes before going to work. After she got out of work she would go down and take the load out of the washer to put into the dryer. Once, when she proceeded to do that, she discovered a whole box of powdered laundry detergent had been spilled inside the washer on top of her clean, wet clothes. We were immediately called downstairs and shown the evidence. Mother thought I had done it, *I, too, thought I must have,* for it was so out of character for Robyn to do such a thing. She finally owned up to it and got a good scolding.

Mother and Dad said we could have a dog, and an ad appeared in the newspaper for a male Pekinese – "Free to a good home." We named 'him' Dixie. *I don't think he ever knew he had a female's name.* He was pretty smart and we taught him many tricks. He could even say, '"Mama!"

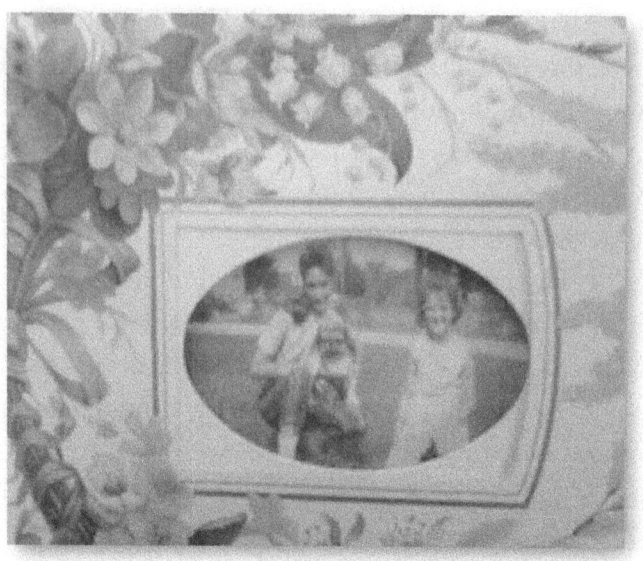

**Left: AKA Amy Kayleen (holding Dixie #1);
right: AKA Robyn Louise.**

Money was still tight and my parents struggled to make ends meet. Each evening, after working all day, before coming home, they would stop at the grocery store and buy food for supper. Still, what we ate every night depended on how good Mother's tips had been that day. She worked at a very nice steak house and gained popularity with the customers there. Mother was well-liked by her boss, too. He would allow her to bring home leftovers from what was scraped off the plates, not for us, but for our pig!

Yes, you heard me right…a pig! Mother had seen a sign while driving on a dirt road one day which read, "Piglets for

Sale." She bought one, put him in the trunk of the car and brought him home; we named him Jimmy. He was so little, but not for long. Below is a picture of little Jimmy and me.

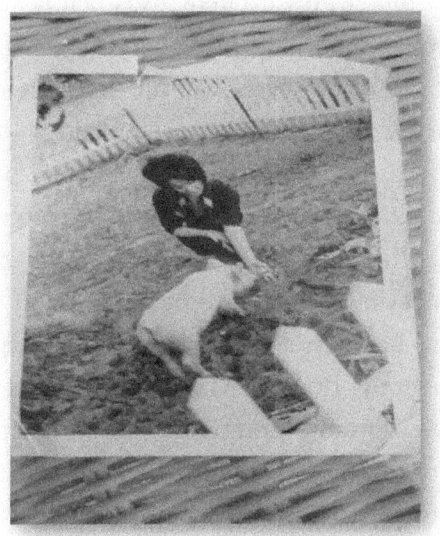

Little Jimmy the pig and me (AKA Amy Kayleen).

Dad built a fence in our backyard and Jimmy ate 'high on the hog' with leftovers from the steak house. Dixie and Jimmy were best of buddies; Jimmy would often mimic Dixie's bark, *I think he thought he was a dog!*

When Jimmy was still young, we brought him into the house just so we could take a picture of him under the Christmas tree. We had that pig for about 3 years at which time, because he had gotten so big, he had to be sold to a local meat processing plant. It took 3 men to wrestle with and get him into the trailer which hauled him away. Mother made a deal for us to get meat in exchange for money, with one stipulation…that it wouldn't be Jimmy!

I'll never forget how excited I was before starting junior high at Hile School. That was the year, 7th grade, when I swallowed a pin in Home Economics class. Not an ink pen, a straight, needle-like pin! The teacher had warned us not to put those things in our mouths, but I didn't pay any attention. *What does she know?* While using the pin to pull stitches from the apron I was sewing, I put it in my mouth for just a minute, bent down to pick something up off the floor and when I raised back up, I took a deep breath and sucked the pin right down my throat! "Mrs. Mark, what would happen if a person swallowed a straight pin?"

"You did what?" That landed me in the nurse's office and a trip to the emergency room. An x-ray was done to 'pinpoint' (*little play on words*) the location, and I was told by the examining doctor to eat bread and celery for the next few days. The thought was the bread and celery would aid in allowing it to pass through my system. *I guess it did, never heard otherwise,* and when the follow-up x-ray was given the pin didn't show up. (News travels fast and often gets misconstrued - Case in point: Someone overheard one of Mother's customer's asking, "Where's Peggy Marie?" Mother's boss replied, "Oh, she's at the hospital, her daughter swallowed a fountain pen!")

That was the same year Mother, Robyn and I went to a thrift store and loaded up on sweaters; they were 10 cents each! We were on cloud nine, as if we had hit the jackpot. One in every color of the rainbow was ours in those second hand sweaters.

Hand me downs continue to exist in my world today. Yard sales and thrift stores are my favorite places to shop, not to mention how packed my house is with things that I just like. (I.e. Both shabby and elegant home-style things, framed biblical verses, vintage furniture, antique radios and wrought iron memorabilia, sculptures of houses, unusual artwork, old pictures, pretty vases, baskets, colorful handmade tapestries, and carved out wooden designs are among my keepsakes.) One might think I would be a good candidate for the popular, televised hoarding show, but there is a story for almost everything I possess, and each thing is valuable to me, so I suppose until I finish telling stories that will always be the case.

If I like something, I like it forever more and it's difficult to part with it. Every once in a while I still think back to the night when I had to put all my earthly possessions in a paper bag and leave everything else behind. That's a tough lesson for a little girl.

I was in a crowded store not too long after that night and I made a decision right then and there, "I want my house to have this much stuff in it someday." I'm almost there! It's not that I idolize 'stuff', but I greatly appreciate the material possessions I have, and if someone gives me something, it's almost a guarantee, I'll hold onto it!

That difficult night of long ago must have been even harder for my dear mother's having to do the same. I'll always remember discovering why her paper bag was so much heavier than Robyn's and my bags. Mother had placed the heavy family bible inside her bag. It wasn't until later in life I came to recognize the importance of God's word, and unlike material possessions or an earthly father, it could forever be relied upon.

CHAPTER 4

Oh What a Life!

This beautiful picture was graciously donated to the
author by Alexandra Wisen, Photographer, 2013.

Enough reminiscing, *now where were we…?*

Oh yeah, by the end of 1983, Bill and I encountered an immoral situation (the CEO of that facility was doing cocaine at work and one of my housekeepers brought it to my attention.) That caused us to again step out on faith and leave our jobs. We knew that was not where God would have us stay. Bill said for me to go first and that he would continue working there until the time was right.

That same day, I put in an application at a new life care facility which hadn't yet been built; it was still just a downtown office in Naples. They hadn't even broken ground for what was to be an exclusive upscale community in North Naples which would include a skilled health care facility. The sales team was in the process of selling units, sight unseen.

After a lengthy interview, I was asked by one of the three owners, "If you came to work for us, when would you be able to start?"

My answer, "I would like to visit my mother in Michigan for a couple of weeks since it was 1981 when I last saw her. After that I would be available."

He advised me to take the trip and asked me to come back and see him when I returned. After a two week stay in Michigan, I did just that.

I went back to that downtown office and met again with the owners. I was told, "If you will come to work for us, your pay will be effective the day you left for Michigan to see your mother. Yep, I landed a job that gave me a two-week paid vacation prior to starting! *How cool is that?*

It wasn't long before an Operations Manager was needed and my dear Bill was the man who was hired for the job. Groundbreaking had occurred, apartments were being built on the eighty-seven acres and were being sold at an alarming rate. Bill was busy with construction punch-out and with the goings on of hiring crews to work on the 9- holed executive length golf course that would be on the grounds, as well as hiring inside and outside maintenance workers while waiting for the twenty-one 3-story buildings, to be completed.

Even though I was hired as the executive housekeeper, until the buildings were up there would be no need for that. Therefore, until that time, I became the acting Move-in co-ordinator working closely with the architect and meeting with future residents, helping them to make architectural changes to the apartments prior to their being built. (At that time, we had no real specialized training.)

While on our way to playing an integral part in the success of what would eventually become the first of its kind, Bill and I shared a secretary; each of us had our own golf carts and separate offices in the maintenance building. The 'University of Hard Knocks' taught us to learn by doing. We had many perks, of which we took full advantage, and we made lots of memories. As department heads, we were guests at the company and employee parties, attended staff meetings, and got to partake of all the amenities.

Fine dining at the clubhouse offered us the tastiest foods. I came to love lamb chops, steaks, savory stews, and was most impressed with various seafood entrees which were served in covered dishes, along with fancy hors d' oeuvres, just to name a few. Old-fashioned etiquette when dining in the clubhouse consisted of jackets worn by the men, and on every table were linen napkins and tablecloths. Correct utensils for every course were laid out at each place setting. *Now even though you can't take the southern out of the girl, this southern gal was very impressed!*

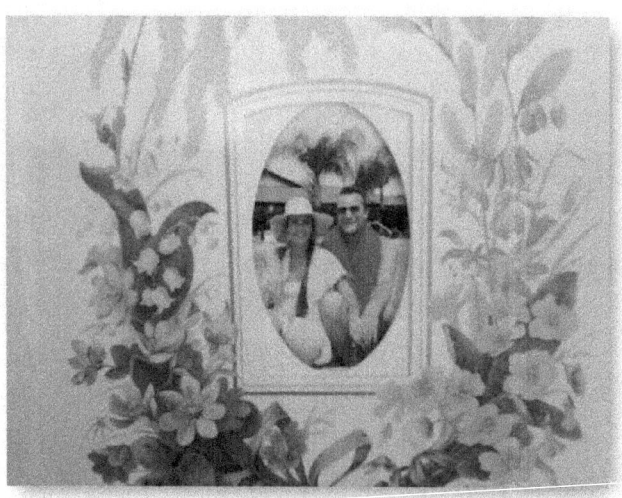

Bill & me (AKA Amy Kayleen) @ company pool party in Naples, Florida (1986).

With company perks come responsibilities and ours were many; the memories we made would forever be engraved in each of our lives. All of our children, at various times, also worked at the facility. We tried always to instill a good work ethic in them by setting a good example.

In 1984, our oldest son took his driving test in the company limousine and passed! I still remember all the people who were at the Secretary of State's office that day, peering out the window, watching him as he parallel parked that stretch limo. That same son, a few years later, came to work for me as the pest control operator. Our other three had jobs in the food service department.

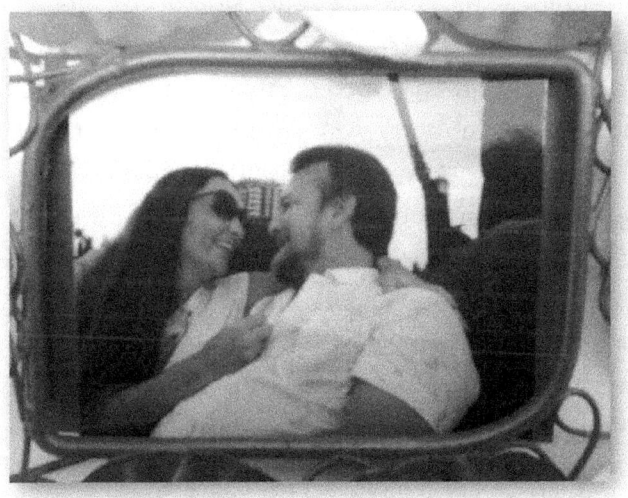

Bill & me (AKA Amy Kayleen). An evening gondola ride on Naples Bay.

By mid-1985, we were able to secure a bank mortgage allowing us to get into our own home (which years prior had been moved onto the lot from the neighboring city of Fort Myers.) It was anchored up on blocks and located in Bonita Springs, a small community on the other side of Naples, just a skip and a jump from our workplace, and not even a mile from the beautiful Gulf of Mexico.

Our modest home was situated on a huge lot, with a shallow creek on one side. In the back yard we had a couple of orange trees and a banana tree, which could be seen when standing on our front deck. Off our back screened-in porch was a kumquat bush, which was handy for making fresh kumquat pie. On the other side of our house was a man-made pond (*I dug and lined it all by myself.*) My dad's brother, Uncle James, helped me make a small waterfall for it while he and Aunt Betty were visiting us one year. The pond was stocked with koi and catfish. The pond's inhabitants helped keep the mosquito population at a minimum.

Shortly after moving there, Bill came home one day and witnessed a group of kids congregated in our driveway, all laughing uncontrollably and pointing toward our deck. When Bill got out of his truck, he immediately heard screaming. One of our sons had dropped his house key between the steps of the deck, and when trying to retrieve it, got his head stuck between the wooden slats. (He had squeezed his head in, but it hadn't dawned on him his ears would get in the way when he tried to pull his head back out.) After a good laugh, Bill took a hammer and pried loose the boards for our son to get free.

Our kids had their own bedrooms, even though they each were jealous of ours. Bill and I shared a 27' long bedroom. (One year when Bill went to Michigan to visit his parents, I singlehandedly installed a laminated wood floor in our room. It turned out great.) We were able to step out onto our screened-in back porch. Complete with candles, it was our little 'getaway!'

Our friends were the people with whom we worked; we were fond of them all. It was nice also to have a surprise visit one year from my forever friend, Jayda Ann. She and her husband came in their motor home and, for a few days, parked in our driveway. We just picked up our conversation where it had left off years prior. However, it was interesting to see we had both grown up, and no longer were we into 'sowing our wild oats'. Instead, we reminisced about all the crazy things in which we had involved ourselves. We were amazed at the realization that God had His hands full making sure we would survive. *It's always good to see her.*

It was handy being close to our work, since Bill was on call 24 hours a day and had to be ready to respond at a moment's notice. He was given a nice, new company truck which had a front and back seat, a trailer hitch, and he was privy to a gas allowance, *nice benefit.* Having the truck allowed us freedom to pull a boat, which an elderly couple from Muskegon kept on our property for us to use. Occasionally, we would hook up the boat trailer to the truck and take the kids fishing in the Gulf. One year our daughter caught an ugly, puffer fish from the back waters of Marco Island. Bill pulled in a catfish and, while trying to get the hook out of its mouth, it flopped around and one of its hard, sharp fins embedded in the side of his foot. Those were the kinds of memories we would often write on postcards to our family and friends who lived back in Muskegon.

I, too, had benefits which came from being a department head. I had assistants who were able to fill in for me if I wasn't there, which was a very good thing. Toward the end of that year, I began experiencing some female problems due to Endometriosis and had to have a complete hysterectomy. Both ovaries were removed and I was started on hormone replacement. It wasn't long before I was back to work. *Enough already!*

No sooner was that over with and hemorrhoids began to be a problem. I had to have surgery for that. *What's going on, here?* Finally, that healed and I was able to resume my busy schedule.

Soon after that, I joined a housekeeping association which helped me tremendously in my job. It was there I learned of a school in Sarasota, which was two hours away, whereby I could obtain credits toward becoming a Certified Executive Housekeeper. It had become apparent to me that more than just good organizational skills were essential for my career. It required me to wear many hats: (i.e. the knowledge of Policies and Procedures, hiring, firing, interviewing techniques, employee training, overseeing and directing cleaning activities, Material Safety Data Sheets, scheduling, budgeting/purchasing, reports, Worker's Compensation laws, customer service and complaints, proper tools and which equipment to order, just to name a few.) Managerial and business experience was definitely a requirement.

I enrolled in the school and began twice a week, after work, making the two hour drive to Sarasota. Two hours in class, then the long drive back home again. Before having play dates with your kids was a popular trend, I tried to have one of them ride with me once in a while. It was a twofold attempt to keep me company, but also to spend some one on one time individually. While I was in class, they were able to do their homework in an adjacent room. They seemed to enjoy it as much as I did, especially the part about stopping half way for a fast food meal.

I always admired Bill's great cooking and clean up skills. Had it not been for his taking on the duties of chief cook and bottle washer, I don't know how we'd have pulled it off. It was always a treat to come home to a clean kitchen and the aroma that had been left behind from a big pot of chili or one of his delicious soups that had simmered for hours on the stove. Whoever hadn't gone with me to Sarasota had a hand in his meal preparation, clean up, and putting away some for the next day's leftovers; he made sure of that.

I put 20,000 miles on my little Ford Escort during the two years I attended the school and achieved a Certified

Executive Housekeeping degree. After that I began taking classes through the mail, completed C.E.U.s (Continuing Education Units) and obtained a Registered Executive Housekeeping degree. Hard work had paid off and, though exhausted, I was at the top of my game.

It was important to the residents that the housekeepers speak English at all times when cleaning apartments. Most of my staff were Hispanic and since I was not bilingual I arranged to have a teacher from the local Vocational Technical Center to come in on my employees' lunch hour and teach them English. It was well received by staff and residents alike.

*I was so proud of my staff and wanted to show them special recognition for all their cooperation and hard work so I started what I called, The Yellow Rose Award. One employee was selected among all the rest and honored for overall performance and attendance. It gained the attention of the news media, and a reporter came out and did an article on me, as well as the selected Yellow Rose recipient. The write-up stated that I had achieved educational credits and was a Registered Executive Housekeeper.

The article received attention from other Executive Housekeepers in the surrounding area who began calling me and inquiring as to how they could obtain classes for themselves. I shared with them what I had done with traveling back and forth to Sarasota. Most all of them said they would be unable to do that.

One day, I decided to stop in at the local Vocational Technical Center just to thank the Director who had so graciously allowed for my employees to receive training. It was during that meeting with him I suggested he arrange for an Executive Housekeeping class to start there and told him about the night classes I had taken.

He thought it was a great idea and, to my surprise, said, "You are right, and I've got just the perfect teacher, you!"

Twice a week, for two and a half years, in addition to my day job, after work in the evenings, I taught the Executive Housekeeping curriculum at that Vocational Technical Center. It was attended by many who worked in the hospitality industry. The pay was excellent.

By 1991, the life-care facility was up and running strong. My title was Director of Housekeeping/Laundry Services. I had a large staff of housekeepers who were busy with construction cleaning apartments that were being built. In addition, residential housekeepers were scheduled on a weekly basis to clean occupied apartments, clubhouses and offices. Finally, the skilled nursing facility took off and I had housekeepers to clean that. My responsibilities had included designing the laundry facility, then overseeing a laundry staff which provided weekly laundry for the apartment residents and health care facility rooms. In addition to all that, I was responsible for overseeing inside pest control. I was one busy lady! *Looking at all that in black and white, I can hardly believe so much was accomplished.*

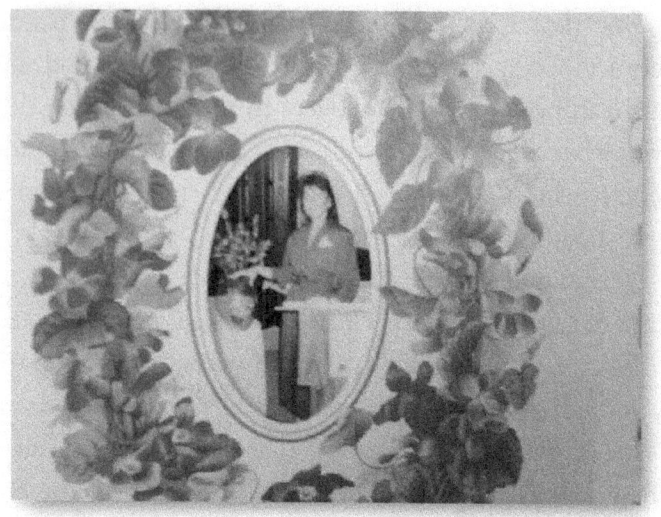

"Executive Housekeeper" me (AKA Amy Kayleen).

In August of that year, during a self-exam, I found a small lump in the side of my left breast and was scheduled to have an excisional biopsy. A surgical procedure was scheduled whereby the doctor removed a small, benign cyst. *Whew! Glad that's over with! I don't have time for this.* As a preventative precaution I began having mammograms yearly.

We kept our Sunday mornings and Wednesday evenings free, for church. Hard as we tried, raising 4 teenagers was no easy task, especially while trying to hold down full time jobs and all the extras that were included. The blended family that we were produced even more obstacles, and we faced challenges at every turn, anywhere from school work to discipline problems. I know we made a lot of mistakes, but we did the best we knew how. No books existed at that time on raising our kind of family. *We wouldn't have had time to read them, anyway! However, I did keep a bible sitting on my desk at work and referred to it daily.*

We had new additions. Everyone in our family of six enjoyed our energetic little dog who was a Boston bull terrier named Gizmo, the large 180 gallon salt water indoor aquarium which was in our Florida room, and the small 25 gallon fresh water fish tank in our living room.

Gizmo was like one of the kids and he provided all of us with much entertainment. He hated frogs! One evening, we were all sitting on the front deck and one hopped over and landed on Gizmo; it covered his whole face. Of course, we all laughed, but he wasn't amused. The frog's feet were like little suction cups on Gizmo's wet nose and stuck to him like glue. After that, he hid whenever he heard the word 'frog.'

After supper one evening, our youngest son said he was going to ride his bike over to see a friend. He went out the back door and within a few seconds ran back into the house; his eyes were as big as saucers, and all color had drained from his face. When he finally was able to speak he said when he went to throw his leg over to get on the bicycle he looked down and there was a snake coiled around the seat.

Needless to say, there was never a dull moment at our house. Saturdays consisted of giving Gizmo a bath, cleaning one or both fish tanks, doing up laundry, shopping for and preparing food for the week ahead. The kids were given specific chores which had to be followed to the max if they were expecting a weekly allowance. We butted heads occasionally but, for the most part, they were pretty good kids. Aside from church outings, an hour or two at the Gulf was usually squeezed into the mix somewhere during the week. I did many bible studies sitting in a lounge chair while soaking in the sun on the shoreline of Bonita Beach.

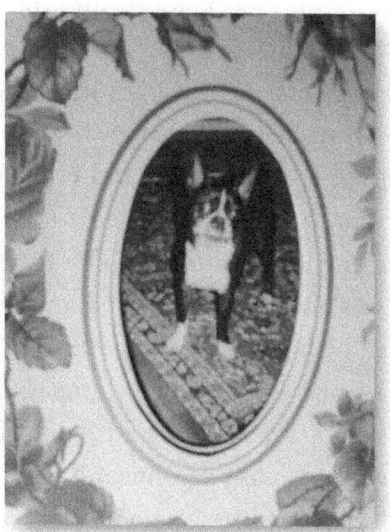

Gizmo

At least three times a week, I would use my lunch hour, change from my work clothes into my bathing suit, and drive to Bonita Beach where I'd walk the water's edge, which was very therapeutic. It was easy and relaxing to let my long hair down, allowing it to be blown by the warm and gentle

Florida breeze if only for a little while, *and is a great way to pray!*

Then, I would pull my hair in place again and secure it with pins after a quick change back into my work apparel and return to my office just in time for a scheduled meeting or routine business. Occasionally Bill and I would sneak off for a little 'sand date' in the middle of the day. It was good for us to enjoy each other that way.

<u>*ABOUT A HOUSEKEEPER…</u>
Housekeeping is something nobody notices, unless it goes undone.
It's a job that's very secure, and the rewards are next to none.
Unless you put it in its proper perspective, it's not a lot of fun.
But, oh what a joy, when you're responsible for a job well done.
A smile of appreciation will send a housekeeper on her way
But a little thank you can brighten her day.
Cleanliness is her goal, come what may, uniqueness is her trademark, I'd say.
It's surprising what their eyes do see while cleaning up after you and me.
Day in and day out there she will be cleaning up after you and me.

She's constantly on the lookout for cobwebs, grease and dirt
Looking high, looking low, always on alert.
All the work that she must do certainly is an effort
She must keep safety in her mind so no one will get hurt.
A housekeeper goes through many tests
Treating anyone she meets as if they were a guest.
She labors long and does her best
And when she goes home, she does the rest...she begins again.
(Written by: Kittye Sharron (dedicated to the housekeeping staff in 1986)

CHAPTER 5

My Million Dollar Bill

"He never ran away and stuck by me through thick and thin...what a man! On my darkest days, he's the one who pulls me up."

(QUOTE BY: KITTYE SHARRON)

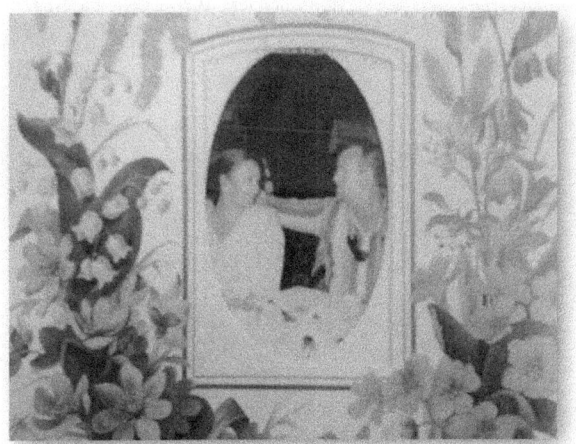

My Million Dollar Bill & me (AKA Amy Kayleen)

My precious husband had been working behind the scenes for all this time and little did I realize how much it had taken its toll on him. Changes were being made at work that caused the department heads much frustration, not to mention the daily responsibilities that were just part of the job.

Bless his heart, he internalized those instances so much that he ended up having an undiagnosed nervous breakdown and he resigned his position. I'm embarrassed to admit, I wasn't very understanding at that time.

"You did what? How are we going to pay all our bills? We've got mouths to feed!"

Bill had called our minister to come over to help me be more compassionate; also some of our church friends came too. *It takes a church to raise a couple!* And it surely took me a while to begin considering what he was experiencing.

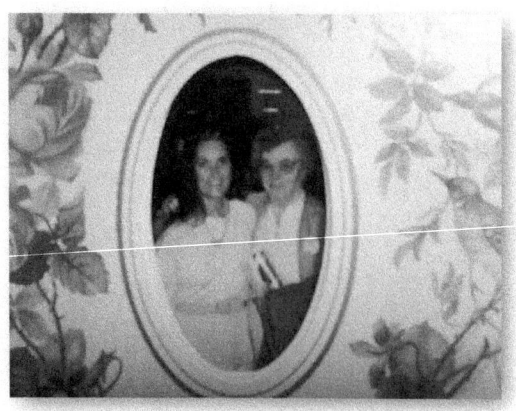

Mama and me (AKA Amy Kayleen)

Things have a way of working out. He ended up doing what he does best…caring for people. Bill took specialized training and began working in a nursing home which was close to our house. Not surprising to me, the people loved him. His gentle spirit and sweet nature had the residents waiting at the door for his shift to begin.

Our house wasn't as full as it had once been. By then, three of our kids were married and had moved away and the youngest one was studying at the community college in Fort Myers.

Of course, we had lost a lot, but it wasn't long before we were blessed beyond belief. Another dear soul came to live with us, my maternal grandmother, Mama. Since my grandfather had died several years before, she had been living alone in a little house in a fruit-farming town way up in Michigan. She had been having little mini strokes and it was not a good idea for her to be alone.

Mama and I had always been close and that stayed the same. When she arrived we just picked up where we had left off. We had so many good times. When I wasn't at work, I took her to the beach with me and we went shopping, reminisced and laughed at the silliest things.

Shortly after Mama came to live with us, being unfamiliar with the terrain, she ended up standing on a fire ant mound while we were at the outdoor flea market. In spite of using all the suggested remedies, that poor thing itched so badly from the many fire ant bites. One Sunday, while she was sitting in church, her leg itched so much that she began to scratch hard enough to rock the entire pew. She couldn't help it. The two of us started laughing, and I thought we were going to draw attention from the entire congregation. *Yes, another church story; as you've already heard, I've had experiences like this before!* Thankfully, her ant bites finally did heal.

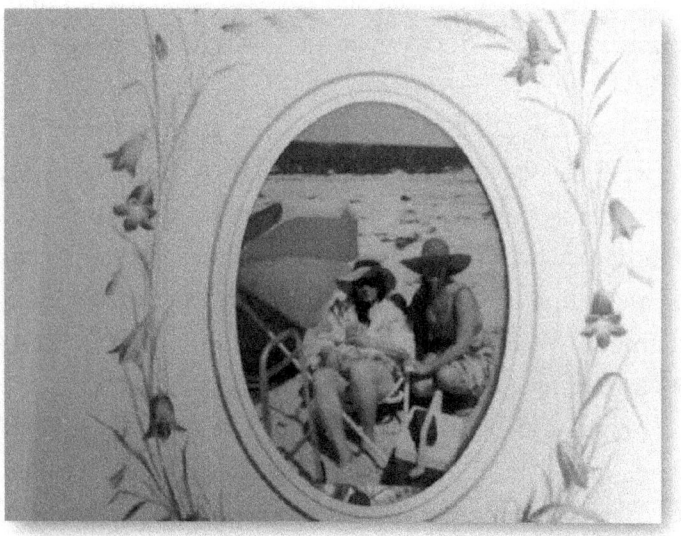

Beach buddies, with walker in tow. (Mama and me at Bonita Beach.)

After the first year and a half, she was confined to a walker and wasn't able to do much but provided me with her sweet company while Bill worked the night shift. She would watch me embroider different colored roses on a yellow tablecloth, which I had bought for a quarter at a yard sale. It seemed like yesterday when as a little girl I sat next to her watching as she embroidered pillowcases. *Now, she watched me.*

During the day, when I was at work, my million dollar Bill cared for Mama until I got home. Then, when it was time for his shift to begin, he went off to work with no complaint.

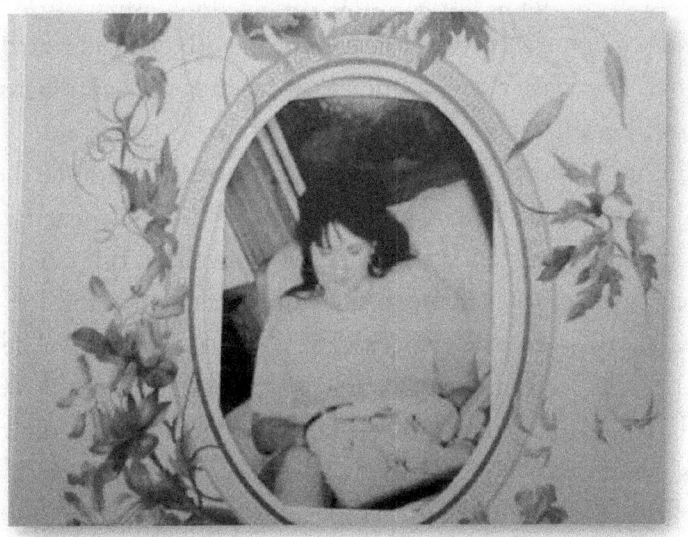

Picture of me (AKA Amy Kayleen) in 1988, when I first began to embroider the yellow tablecloth. Finished it 24 years later; that picture is shown near the back of the book.

Gizmo loved Mama; she always fed him part of her supper when I wasn't looking. Then Bill would give candy to Mama when I wasn't looking. She wasn't supposed to have very many sweets but she loved them and would charm Bill into making sure he didn't forget about her. Of course, he didn't give her a lot, but she thought he did; he meant the world to her.

Because Mama had such a difficult time getting in the bathtub, our ½ bathroom had a walk-in shower which was where she would bathe. One year when Robyn and my brother-in-law came for a visit, Robyn and I thought it would feel good to Mama to have a tub bath. She did enjoy it; however, when it came time to get her out of the tub, we had a terrible time. She wasn't strong enough to use her legs and arms to push herself up, and we couldn't lift her. Mama said, "Get Bill; he'll know what to do; he'll get me out!" And, he did.

Mama's health began to take its toll and eventually she was unable to stand, not even with a walker. Bill cared for her, dressed and bathed her, combed her hair, took her on walks using a wheelchair and would put a hat on her head. Then the two of them would busy themselves in the yard. He would hand her the hose and she would water my roses while he mowed the grass. Gizmo would be right at her wheels. Occasionally, she would spray him with the hose and her laughter would explode as he, standing next to her, shook off the water, ran up on the deck, then back again for more.

Mama went to be with the Lord in 1995. I learned so much from her down through the years; at the end of her life, she taught me how to die. I don't know who took it hardest, but through my own tears I watched my dear Bill cry like a baby when she took her last breath. Gizmo was never the same after that and he, too, died of epilepsy not long after Mama passed.

Sadly, while Mama was alive, I didn't get to finish my yellow tablecloth, but 24 years later I did. (Picture of finished tablecloth in the back of the book.)

Excerpt from The Longest Letter: Incredible Hope: *"It will be a beautifully unique tapestry, woven with threads of many colors and, like her, will always hold a special place in the garden of my heart."*

Mama's death never gets any easier and, while the world spins, I am still grief stricken; my heart still mourns. Certain smells, sounds, and sights still trigger the memory of my sweet grandmother. (I.e. Pineapple Upside Down cake, seeing someone with lightly permed hair, old recipes, beautiful handwriting, or her favorite snack, a red, Delicious apple.)

After Mama was gone, and our youngest son went off to college in another state, it was just too quiet at our house. I found an ad in the paper advertising another Boston bull terrier and, like I did with Gizmo, paid $500 for Caleb. When not quite a year old, he ended up following Bill out the door one day, ran in the street and got hit by a car. Poor Bill ran out to the road, scooped him up, brought him in the house, and began giving him mouth to mouth resuscitation, to no avail. Bill was devastated.

That Bill was so down that the next day he went to the dog pound and brought home this flea bitten, mixed breed of a mutt who was loaded with ticks.

"Why did you get her?"

"Well," he said, "I just asked them which one they were going to put down today and she was it!"

Poor girl was in such bad shape, the fleas and ticks had, literally, chewed holes in her ears. While she laid on the porch, Bill at one end, I at the other, using tweezers and rubbing alcohol, pulled countless ticks off her. Then Bill carried her, put her into the bathtub and together we got her cleaned up. That sweet doggie smelled so good when we were done and she seemed so appreciative; it was easy to love her. That's how we got our Dixie girl! (Named after the Pekinese dog I had growing up, only *this time Dixie was indeed a female.*)

One of the residents at the life care facility had a little black pug which became too mischievous for her to handle; she was looking for a good home for him. That's how we ended up with our Biscuit boy. It took a spray bottle with water to train him to obey.

Dixie and Biscuit became best buddies; Dixie was Bill's and Biscuit was mine. We all had each other. At the time, I didn't realize just how much Biscuit was indeed mine and the marvelous gift he obviously had.

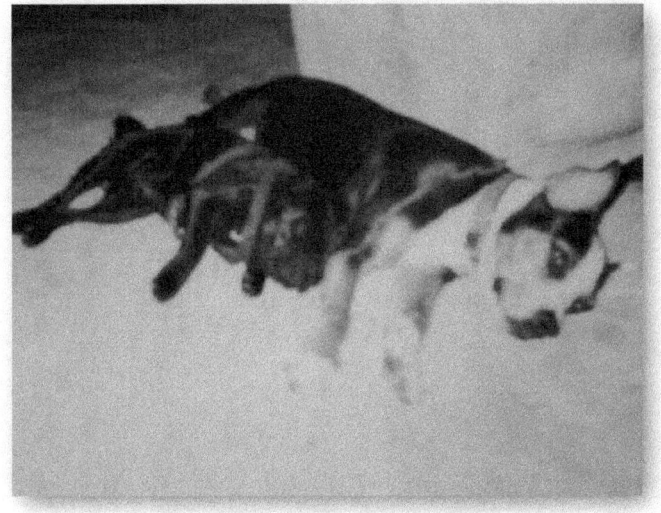

Best buddies: Biscuit & Dixie #2

CHAPTER 6

Our World Turns Upside Down

DUE TO AN OLD INJURY, Bill had to have corrective sinus surgery; a piece of bone had to be taken out of his hip to be used in his forehead where the bone had died. After the surgery he ended up developing MRSA (Methicillin resistant Staphylococcus aureus: a strain of bacteria which is resistant to powerful antibiotics!) which started in his hip. He was put in isolation. After many rounds of antibiotics, it still wouldn't heal. He had to be put on intravenous antibiotics for over 6 months, and he had to wear gloves and a mask. Of course, he couldn't work. Finally, it was cured with a combination of antibiotics.

His only sister, who lived in Michigan, had just been diagnosed with stage 4 pancreatic cancer and needed help. Since Bill had been off work for so long, once he became noncontagious, he went to Michigan to help her and was there until she passed away.

His grandmother, Nan, was also on her death bed in Michigan. It was good that Bill was there to help his mother care for her, too, during that time.

The pressures were only just beginning. I'm not sure exactly when it started, but I was having a difficult time concentrating and noticed I was, more often than not, unable to focus on reading reports. Too, I was having overall, chronic pain which interrupted my sleep and work, and I was experiencing extreme fatigue. The doctor diagnosed me as having Fibromyalgia.

By 1999, it had become so debilitating, that the doctor had put me on permanent disability. I resigned my dream job. Bill returned home and we put the house on the market. The first people who came to look at it bought it. We were on our way to live back to where we had moved from 18 years earlier. *Once again, God's amazing grace had changed our hearts and our circumstances.*

With Nan's passing, we inherited her house in Muskegon, Michigan. I didn't put two and two together at that time, but when we were living in Florida we had a house payment. *The Lord had it arranged that we now had a home that was paid for in Michigan. He knows our needs before we even ask!*

One night, in the summer of 2000, I was sitting in my easy chair with my feet propped up. Biscuit started putting his cold nose on my warm left leg.

"Stop that, Biscuit!"

I quickly pulled the light weight afghan over my legs, at which time he immediately began pushing his nose closer to my leg; same spot.

"Biscuit!" I scolded.

Over the next few days he continued sniffing and trying to weasel up to my left leg. Since I was dealing with the discomfort of Fibromyalgia I had failed to take notice that I was actually having pain in that leg, so much so that it was unbearable to put weight on it. I went to the doctor who ordered a Doppler scan. It showed I had a blood clot in the calf of my leg. That Biscuit had been able to smell that with his little pug nose!

In addition to that, I was having trouble breathing. The technician, in all her wisdom, suggested I call that to my doctor's attention. Sure enough, a test was ordered which showed blood clots in both my lungs, too. I was admitted to the hospital on complete bedrest and was started on blood thinners.

Regular doctor visits and mammograms, just to make sure I was all right, became routine. Except for an occasional urinary tract infection, always preceded by a vaginal odor and treated with antibiotics, tests of that nature always came back normal.

I had started talking to a Christian counselor who had really helped me in dealing with what had happened to me as a child. (A later chapter, My Little Girl Book, will reveal an exercise which enabled me to put that horrible memory to rest.) Between his council and that of my physician, I was at that time, diagnosed with Post Traumatic Stress Disorder (PTSD.)

In 2003, I began having to clear my throat often, coughing a lot, and my voice was hoarse. Upon referral, the ENT (Ear, Nose, Throat, Head & Neck,) Dr. Paul Lomeo, D.O. looked into my throat. Then he used a scope, which entailed putting a tube into my nostril and down my throat; he told me I had something called Lingual Tonsils, "But that's not the worst part!" he said. *One never wants to hear a doctor say that!*

Sleep apnea was just one of the diagnoses which future tests would show. It could be helped by the use of a CPAP machine. But, Dr. Lomeo was right, there was a worse part; I had complete airway obstruction, and a huge tumor on the right carotid artery which, of course, would require surgery. However, before that could be done, a Tracheotomy had to be performed to allow an open airway for the removal of the tumor.

So, for the next few months, I had a hole in my neck with a tube sticking out that had to be suctioned regularly, home oxygen, aerosol compressor, a nebulizer and a hospital bed, all in the comfort of my living room.

The carotid artery tumor was removed in 2005; it was benign. *Praise The Lord!*

In 2006, I was hospitalized for Pneumonia, at which time the doctors performed a nuclear scan of the abdominal area and discovered evidence of five, small calcified lymph nodes believed to be accessory spleens. *C'mon, what's going on?*

In 2007, excessive coughing required more surgery, the scraping of benign lingual tonsil growths from my throat.

In 2008, a benign growth had to be removed from my big toe along with the correction of a heel spur in my left foot.

The gynecologist had to administer more antibiotics due to chronic urinary tract infections, then remove a benign vaginal cyst in 2009. It was at that time I was diagnosed with Interstitial Cystitis (chronic pelvic pain/spasms/nerve ending pain.) I was also put on an estrogen cream and a tablet to be used vaginally twice a week.

Also, that same year, I had to have cataract surgery in both eyes, with lens implants.

The year of 2010 produced more challenges. A benign ganglionic cyst was removed from my right middle finger. Toward the end of the year, the left side of my neck became bothersome, and further testing revealed it was a cancerous lymph node.

In 2011, Thyroid cancer reared its ugly self; a Para ganglia was removed from my left carotid artery. After that, I received Radioactive Iodine Treatment in the form of six huge pills that had to be swallowed. *The rest of my life I will need to take a thyroid supplement and have regular blood testing to monitor Thyroid Stimulating Hormone (TSH.)*

I continued to have regular mammograms but, in 2012, calcification was detected in the left breast. A chip was inserted to mark the area so that each time a mammogram was done that area could be monitored closely.

It was during one of the mammograms the machine was squeezing me so tightly it caused a discharge from my right nipple. When I questioned the technician she explained there had probably been a little fluid-filled cyst that had ruptured. The discharge continued from the right nipple and over time became a sore that bled and wouldn't heal. The gynecologist thought it was an irritated duct and he said we'd watch it.

In September a needle biopsy was done on my left breast and it was determined that the calcification detected earlier was benign.

That same year I had to undergo treatment at the bladder clinic for a couple of months for pain in my bladder. I was told at that time that some microscopic blood had been detected during a urine test, but it didn't seem to be too much of a concern for the gynecologist.

In the year 2013, more benign lingual tonsils were removed. *I was told this will be something that will need to be done every so often because they will continue to come back.*

The bleeding from my right nipple was still going on. My gynecologist referred me to a surgeon, who also thought it was just an irritated duct. He said to watch it for 6 months and if not any better to come back and see him. Too, another mammogram was done; no sign of cancer.

During that time, abdominal pain, and some vaginal itching and burning, was also present. I continued weekly treatment at the bladder clinic.

By 2014, the surgeon finally decided to do a biopsy on my right nipple. When the results came back, he called me at home. *I always dread a home-call from the doctor, it's never a "hi how are you!" and his call was no different.*

Results: Cancer, stage 1 – Ductal carcinoma in situ of right breast.

I was given a few options (i.e. single, partial or double mastectomy; or remove just the nipple, or the nipple and the areola…OR seek a second opinion.) *What to do? Oh, my!*

My prayer, "Lord, send me a miracle doctor."

The next day, the phone rang. It was a sweet friend from church who was herself a surgical assistant at our local hospital. She suggested I see a Surgical Oncologist in Grand Rapids by the name of Dr. Marianne Melnik, MD, FACS. I didn't waste any time. The Lord has worked through people before and I was certain He had used my friend to get the message to me.

I was able to make an appointment that same week, which was a good thing, but negative self-talk didn't help me to feel better. *Must not be that great; everybody knows a good doctor is hard to get in to see! Might as well go through with it; after all, what have I got to lose?*

A woman feels like less of a woman when faced with problems of this kind. Bill knew just what to say to reverse my thoughts. "I'd love you even if that hole between your legs was sewn together!" (Made me laugh, then made me realize just how blessed I was. As off-colored as his comment had been, with those words my husband had assured me he would love me through it all. *What a man!*)

I was banking on that reassurance as we drove into that huge parking garage in the busy city of Grand Rapids and was thankful for the parking ticket that came out of the machine. *Good thing it has a number on it to remind us where we are parked.* The building towered over the others in that downtown metropolis. Granite lined the glass elevator floor; and a most impressive décor came into view as the doors opened and Bill and I stepped off onto the 4th floor. Huge space allowed one to peer over the railing and look down to the floors below, a beautiful view; I was lost in the moment. *How will we ever find our way out of this massive place?*

But that was the least of my concerns. As I registered, filled out forms, and waited impatiently for my name to be called, I remembered the prognosis. Needless to say, I was plagued with many emotions and in my mind had myself, over and over again, dead and buried.

I found myself watching Bill as he sat there peacefully reading a magazine and acting as though he didn't have a care in the world. *I only wish I could be so relaxed!* I silently prayed, "Lord, I'm straddling faith and fear; help me to know that my breasts do not define me, rather, you do."

I heard my name called and the nurse motioned, "Right this way."

As if very brave, standing erect, I straightened my shoulders and smiled as I walked in the direction of the voice of the one holding open the door. *Truth be known, inside I'm like a crumbling cracker, just bits and pieces of once model material; my 66 years had come down to this.*

"Please be seated." She looked over my paperwork, stating the doctor had already received my records from Muskegon. She gave me a half gown and said, "Everything from the waist up take off. Then put this on. The doctor will see you shortly."

When I saw the attractive, petite, young-looking female come into the exam room I was just sure I was in the wrong place, but her name tag had given her away. She shook hands with both Bill and me, Dr. Melnik's manner was as flawless as her complexion. A soft voice came through her painted, coral-colored lips, which exposed pretty white teeth as she smiled. She stood not even 5' tall and had a head full of beautifully arranged dishwater blonde, curly hair. I caught a glimpse of hope in her glistening eyes, but, *she sure doesn't look like a wise ole' doctor!*

It didn't take long for me to realize there was more to her than pearly whites, curly locks and initials behind her name!

CHAPTER 7

Breast Cancer, The Best Thing That Ever Happened to Me!

AFTER EXAMINING ME, DR. MELNIK said, "Considering what you have been through, I would suggest you have Genetic Testing." *What's that?*

With Bill and me looking on in desperation, she explained her suspicions: the possibility of a hereditary link might well be responsible for the rare occurrences of my medical past. She was especially interested in my history of the Pheochromocytoma tumor that had been found in 1974.

"I see no reason why you would have to have anything but the cancerous nipple and areola removed from your right breast; no need for anything more." *My mind is at ease.*

She gained my trust and, by the following month, August, 2014, Dr. Melnik had performed surgery on me, removing only the nipple and areola from my right breast, followed up by a good report. All the cancer in the right breast was gone; none in the lymph nodes. *Yay!* Furthermore, she referred me to a Plastic Surgeon who would be able to reconstruct the areola and nipple. *Wonderful!*

Additionally, blood work was ordered for the genetic test that she seemed so adamant about my getting and, upon her advice, Bill and I were scheduled to meet with the Genetic department, which was located in the same building.

Along with the bloodwork, the procedure consisted of filling in multiple pages of family history and having an initial appointment with a genetic doctor and counselor. It was as if I had been rescued from a sinking ship. Those two women that were in that department, Dr. Judith Hiemenga, MD (Clinical Geneticist) and the Genetic Counselor, Mary Mobley, MS, CGC, took an interest in me and did not act like I was crazy. *Bless their hearts!*

The waiting game is a difficult one to play and I was so appreciative during that time to know I was being prayed for. In fact, that's where my strength came from. I was encouraged daily by sweet cards and messages from family and friends.

Jayda Ann was one who reached out to express her concern. *Time has changed both of us for the better. We still stay in touch online, and see each other every so often; I tell her she has evolved to become 'a blessed blast from my past!'*

As always, my Mother and sister were especially helpful while I was trying to whittle away the weeks. I don't know what I would have done without their life-giving words and heartfelt talks which often took place into the night; not to mention the food they made just for me. Both of them have the gift of hospitality, *which was, and still is, bestowed on me over and over again. (Among other things, my sister is famous for her potato rolls; my mother makes the world's greatest fried chicken, also chicken and dumplings, biscuits and cornbread dressing.) My mother and my sister mean the world to me.*

Bill and I would often meet my mother, my stepfather, Robyn, and her husband, at a favorite quaint little restaurant in Muskegon; *it continues to be a meeting place for all of us.* It's called Herbies Café, where breakfast is served until they close at 2:00 p.m. Robyn says they fry her eggs just the way she likes them and my brother-in-law loves their sausage gravy over a southern omelet, which they will prepare according to your specifications. Actually, I'm fond of their biscuits and the fact that the coffee in your cup never gets cold; when down about an inch a friendly waitress is there to fill it again. Too, they serve one of my old time favorites, a hot beef sandwich with brown gravy. My stepfather usually has blueberry pancakes and Mother likes their breakfasts and their blackberry jelly. There is nothing fancy about Herbies, just a home atmosphere which brings me back to the memories of the days of long ago when a good meal was shared and everybody knew your name, or at least recognized your face. *There they still do!*

Of course, my children and grandchildren provided me, *still do,* with sincere, loving, thought-filled words of encouragement during those waiting days. Knowing I was nestled in their prayers kept me afloat as I drifted in what seemed to be a sea of uncertainty. It was, *and continues to be*, a blessing to receive a card or message from them or different ones in their church family telling me I was being lifted in prayer. Sometimes when we don't know how to pray, someone else does; *I consider that a resource, a source of strength.*

Bill, my man of few words, always knew when I was having a weak moment. He was, *and continues to be*, my rock. He went then *and continues to go* to every doctor's appointment with me, asked questions that I didn't think of, understood the medical jargon and explained all to me in language I could understand. Often, without a word, *he just knows when to put his arm around me and what to say, usually nothing, but is there to comfort me, day or night, doesn't matter! He gives me a smile and a touch which goes straight to my heart!*

By the end of October, five weeks had passed, and the test results were back. Again, Bill and I met with the genetic counseling team to go over the findings indicated, in part, below:

RESULTS: POSITIVE: PATHOGENIC MUTATION DETECTED. This individual is heterozygous for the p.W200C pathogenic mutation in the SDHB gene. The result is consistent with a diagnosis of hereditary paraganglioma-Pheochromocytoma (PGL/PCC) syndrome. Cancer risk estimate: lifetime risks of 77-100% for paragan-

glioma-Pheochromocytoma and up to 14% for renal cell carcinoma (RCC) ++. The expression and severity for this individual cannot be predicted. Genetic counseling is a recommended option for all individuals undergoing genetic testing.

MY (not so savvy) INTERPRETATION after reading the report and meeting with the genetic team: I have a rare, highly hereditary, mutated gene that is identified as SDHB (Succinate dehydrogenase complex, subunit B.) *(If you want to read more about it, get on your computer and google in: SDHB.)* Among other things, the SDHB gene mutation puts me at a higher risk for cancer; it is linked to various cancers (thyroid, breast, kidney,) benign growths, and is connected to Paraganglioma/Pheochromocytoma syndrome.

Any and all doctors who provide treatment for me need to be aware of this: Preventative testing needs to occur regularly which will consist of, but not limited to, CT scans for early detection of any new occurrences. Any and all growths that develop need to be closely monitored and biopsied without delay.

Also, all three of my sons need to be tested to see if this gene has been passed on to them. If it has, my grandchildren run the risk of having inherited it. Additionally, my sister and half-brother need to be tested to determine whether they carry the mutated gene. The strange part in all of this is, one doesn't necessarily need to have symptoms in order to carry the mutation and/or pass it on.

The genetic team concluded one in a million people have this and very likely I had inherited the SDHB mutated gene from my deceased father. *What are the chances I would be that one in a million? What are the chances my sister would be? My sons? My half-brother? My grandchildren? My extended family?*

Once again I had, what seemed to be, an unsurmountable task; to let my loved ones know that they, too, if related to my biological father, needed to be tested. I felt as though my family must surely think I was a fanatic or that it was all in my head. *Perhaps it was my approach, or maybe the content of the message…*"You've got to get tested!" *"Hey, I know you don't want to hear this, and, I haven't been trained how to get the word out, but I've been told to pass this information on to my family! Believe me, this is not something I chose, I was born with it! And, since you are in my family you might have been born with it, too! Oh, and one other thing, your doctor probably won't know anything about it and more than likely will have never heard of SDHB!" (Lord, I think you need to send another messenger, I'm not a very good one.)*

I learned that it is extremely important to find a doctor or clinical center with extensive experience in Pheochromocytoma, paraganglioma and the management of patients with the SDHB gene. Not everyone with the mutation will develop tumors or end up with metastatic Pheo/paraganglioma, but the risk seems to be much greater with SDHB. Therefore, it's important to know if the mutated gene is in your body. It's not a death sentence; some people who have received proper treatments have been known to live long lives. However, there are others who have had a very aggressive form and are totally unaware of the root cause. While there is no cure for a genetic mutation, there is screening and testing in place which is useful in detecting these tumors so that treatment can be appropriately administered. More is being learned about SDHB every day by wonderful researchers who are very committed to studying it and trying to help patients.

My primary physician in Muskegon, Dr. Ogas, encouraged me to talk to my sons and convince them to be tested. He was adamant about it. Frantically, I began running copies of the results from the genetic testing that had been done on me and distributing to my family. *"Don't pooh, pooh this! It may affect you or your children! True, you may not have symptoms, but you may still have this hereditary mutated gene; please read and take this to your doctor, and ask him/her to request genetic testing for you. SDHB isn't something that will show up in a routine blood test; it must be specially ordered. This is a matter of life or death! Don't be a fool, I'm trying to save your life!" They must think I'm crazy!* I probably sounded like Chicken Little, "The sky is falling!"

Memories of my father resurfaced in my mind as I thought back to how much he would perspire. No doubt, he, too, had carried and passed along to me, when I was conceived, the SDHB mutated gene and he had no way of knowing. The perspiring is only one of many symptoms, (we were the lucky ones! Not!) *I don't think my family understands that not everyone who has the genetic mutation will perspire as my dad and I did.* SDHB is linked to Pheochromocytoma, but not everyone with the SDHB gene mutation will have Pheochromocytoma; however, they may have other things going on which could be detrimental to their existence. *It is unknown now as to who else in the family had been or will be affected, and we don't know for sure where it began.*

As I dug deeper into my memory bank I realized that this daughter's quest to avenge her father's murder would, instead, best be served determining why he died. I am convinced it was due, in part, to a hereditary link. His father, my paternal grandfather, had a huge growth on his neck (possibly thyroid cancer and/or a paraganglioma.) An old country doctor had said it was a goiter, but not much was known back in those days about genetics. Too, he had been diagnosed to have prostate and lung cancers. After a careful review, I think he was a carrier of the highly hereditary, SDHB mutated gene, and that it was passed down to my father, me, and only God knows who else in our extended family. One of my dad's sisters is in failing health and, since she has had Para ganglia benign growths and various problems, it is suspected she, too, carries the mutated gene. Some of my paternal uncles and cousins have also had various cancers.

In an effort to further understand the dangers all of us who carry this gene mutation might be facing, I have recently learned that there are hidden truths regarding SDHB carriers and the use of alcohol (even smoking); it's akin to stepping on a landmine. For those who carry the SDHB mutation, alcohol consumption and smoking are known to intensify blood pressure, speed up the heart, cause a deficiency of oxygen, and an increase of anxiety and adrenalin levels which can lead to a heart attack, stroke and/or death. **Pieces of the puzzle began to fall into place; I believe the gene that stumped the doctors ultimately killed my dear father. (Newsflash: In looking back over my bad choices, I realize now, it could have been me!)**

Thankfully, some in my family began to listen.

To date, my half-brother, my niece, and some of my paternal cousins are planning to be tested; especially since **two of my sons, my sister, my nephew and, my two grandsons were tested and diagnosed with the SDHB gene mutation and,** *each one of them has had their own set of circumstances. How rare is that? According to DNA, it's only a matter of time before others in my family and extended family may begin to show signs related to this. Fortunately, my other son and two of my granddaughters tested negative.*

My dear sister has already had numerous health issues including: battling breast and kidney cancers; a benign Para ganglia on her thyroid; she has had numerous benign growths; and a pre-cancerous pancreatic cyst was discovered during a preventative CT scan, which was removed before it could advance to her lymph nodes. (To date, she has not had a Pheochromocytoma tumor.) Her doctors, too, have had to learn from her.

I was honored the following year when asked by the genetic specialists if I would be willing to speak at the hospital to third year medical students about my SDHB gene mutation and how it had affected me. The first thing I told those students was to 'listen.' I encouraged them to not give up on patients with confusing symptoms that sounded preposterous; it may not be in their heads, rather in their genes.

The hospital even arranged for me to be interviewed and a write-up was done on my case and appeared in their widely circulated medical newsletter which spoke about DNA (stands for: deoxyribonucleic acid, which is the molecule that carries genetic information in humans and all other living organisms.)

Furthermore, my condition was so rare that I was asked to participate in a nationwide study at a famous medical hospital/clinic. *Indeed, I am involved in that.*

I am convinced that I am alive today because of genetic testing. With so many medical anomalies over the years: numerous benign growths, including the Pheochromocytoma tumor, thyroid and breast cancers, *I'm just glad my kidneys are okay!* **Really?** (That would prove to be short lived, **I should not have been so quick to make that assumption!**) *READ ON…!*

CHAPTER 8

Microscopic No More

For the last several years, I had been told microscopic blood was showing up in my urine cultures. What I couldn't see hadn't caused me any real concern, but the morning I went to the bathroom and saw actual blood droplets in the toilet, I became greatly concerned. I called the gynecologist's office.

I was told to come in for a urine test immediately. Once at the office, after the urine test, the nurse said she would squeeze me in to see the doctor since I didn't have an actual appointment. Sure enough, that would prove beneficial.

He said a urine culture would be done which would take a few days to get back, and he prescribed antibiotics for me to start on for he was fairly sure the results would show a urinary tract infection. However, when I mentioned that I had recently been told to alert all my doctors about the SDHB mutation, surprisingly, he told me he had never heard of it. He got on his computer right then and, after reading the description, referred me to be seen by the Urologist; an appointment was made for the following week.

Am I in the right place? The urologist, too, was unfamiliar with SDHB and he too got on his computer right there in the exam room. On that day, January 13th, 2015, he ordered a CT scan of my abdomen and he said it should take a few days for the results. I would be getting a call from his office staff when the results were back.

By the 20th I hadn't heard anything from the urologist's office, (*no news is good news*), but was excited for my outpatient, surgical procedure being done that day by the Plastic Surgeon. My right breast was reconstructed using no foreign tissue, rather my own body fat. Too, I was so pleased because both breasts received a lift which would make them symmetrical. Even the nipple was reconstructed. *Amazing what they can do nowadays!*

Once I was released, Bill, my mother and I, while riding back home from the hospital in Grand Rapids, were each expressing how glad we were that the surgery was over and it was all downhill from here on in. *Really?*

No sooner had we walked in the doorway of our home, the phone rang, and it was the Urologist. *Just to say, hello? No, of course not!*

RESULT of CT SCAN of my ABDOMEN: CANCEROUS TUMOR in RIGHT KIDNEY.

The urologist went on to say my right kidney was going to have to come out. The size of the tumor practically took up my entire kidney. There was no possible way to save it. And, due to my medical history, the surgery would be too complex to perform in Muskegon. He said surgery would need to be done at Ann Arbor's U of M Hospital, and a referral was being made to the kidney specialist there.

On the 3rd of March, 2015, my right kidney was removed. I was told afterward that the cancerous kidney tumor had been there for over a decade. (It was there even before the thyroid and breast cancers!) And, *I have to give credit where credit is due*; that kidney specialist actually called me at home a few days after I was discharged to say, "I just called to see how you are doing!" *Imagine that!*

Because of genetic testing, the tumor was detected and removed before it could spread. It had been contained and did not affect the surrounding lymph nodes. Oh how richly God blesses us with other people. Physical recovery was made possible through the grace of the Lord Jesus. All glory to Him, for He is good.

The following chapters offer some valuable tools that I regularly use. They work for me and are a part of who I am.

CHAPTER 9

My Little Girl Book

I HAD SOME VERY DARK days dealing with painful shame. It was coming from memories of the childhood sexual molestation that had occurred when I was only 8 years old. Though 45+ years had passed, I could not escape the horrific nightmares which would continually creep into the restorative sleep that was lacking in my body.

The Christian counselor suggested I go through an exercise whereby I write a letter from my heart which would never be sent…to my perpetrator, the pedophile, who had long since died.

Beforehand, I thought very seriously as to how I would proceed. I went to the Christian bookstore and thumbed through various journals until I saw it. I felt a connection and I bought 'my little girl book'. The front cover depicted pure innocence. Pictured was a very young girl sitting on the ground wearing a white dress, leaning against a tree, with pen and paper in her hand. The sky behind her was a dark gray, very much like the gloomy colorless nights with which I wrestled.

After praying, I opened the journal and reached for a pen with which to write. It wasn't blue ink or black, it had red ink. I reasoned that would be the perfect choice since the words I would write would be coming from my heart.

As I wrote, the pages of my journal began to be dampened by the tears falling from my eyes. They were tears I never before allowed myself to shed for they had been stuffed so tightly into the grooves of my heart that it actually hurt to cry them.

I continued writing, and spent weeks perfecting that letter. I prayed a lot during that time. With each page I wrote, it was as though I had been peeling an onion. Vivid pictures in my mind's eye began to emerge, and I took a close look at what I had tried to shut out from my mind so many years earlier. Layers upon layers were peeled back, which exposed the sinful acts of my cowardly offender.

It felt as though raw nerves were bleeding and many times I wanted to stop writing. I reminded myself, *this is an exercise; without pain there will be no gain!*

From the deepest darkest caverns of my heart, I dug, shovelful after shovelful piling up the dirty memories of that dark night and throwing them into that letter which was fueled by stored up anger. After weeks of writing, I completely filled that journal. In fact, I fully intended to share some of those writings with you.

However, when I went to look for my journal, I couldn't find it. I looked high and low, even dug through boxes I had packed away, *"Where's my little girl book? I wouldn't have thrown that away."*

No, I didn't throw it away. It was then I remembered the night I had piled kindling loosely into the fire pit on my back porch, then arranged sticks in the shape of a teepee. Days of camping had taught me to slowly blow air into the structure as it was ignited in order to build heat and intensity. I had always enjoyed watching a fire, but that was a bitter sweet night.

Into the flames, I had placed 'my little girl book'. After all those writings and all those tears, I watched as my journal was enveloped by the fire and thought how much those memories had consumed and crippled me for so many years. *Now, they were being burned up.*

No longer did I need to cling to those memories or revisit them over and over again. For in the letter I had also stated I forgave him. I needed to be refined; burning that journal was my way of releasing the pain, the anger, which had kept me bound like a prisoner.

It wasn't meant that I should share those writings. Instead, *I want to share, that I no longer cling to those memories; today I cling to God.* He showed me how to forgive so that I would know how to forgive others. Proverbs 27:17 says that iron sharpens iron, so one person sharpens another. There is mutual benefit in the rubbing of two iron blades together; the edges become sharper, making the knives more efficient in their task to cut and slice. Likewise, the Word of God is a 'double-edged sword" (Hebrews 4:12) and it is with this that we are to sharpen one another.

There was such cleansing in that exercise, for you see, the memory of that painful night had become like a cancerous tumor and needed to be removed, cut out! Purified by fire, the memories burned up, but I was left intact.

"For you have tried us, Oh God; you have refined us as silver is refined." (Psalm 66:10)

CHAPTER 10

Devotions at 3

SINCE MY SPLEEN WAS REMOVED, I have been very susceptible to catching just about any illness that comes my way. In an effort to stay healthy and well, I try to avoid crowded rooms and sitting next to anyone who may have anything contagious. In fact, for that reason, Bill and I try always to sit on the outside of a row, never in the center.

My immune system is compromised because of not having a spleen. Without it, my body lost some of its abilities to produce protective antibodies and to remove unwanted microorganisms from the blood. *As a result, my body's way to fight infection is impaired.*

The spleen is an important organ in the body. It acts as a filter for purifying the blood. Among other things, it produces white blood cells that fight bacteria and infection.

Is it any wonder that when I heard wheezing and deep coughing behind me at church, I cringed? It was coming my way from a little girl who was probably about 8 years old. I'd never seen her before; *must be a visitor.* She was making her way down the aisle followed by her disheveled mother, who was carrying an infant and was also holding the hand of a coughing toddler. *Boy, does she look rough! Oh no, she must have something contagious... oh, please don't let her sit next to me. I don't want to catch her cold, I don't have a spleen!*

Sure enough, the little girl plopped right down in the seat next to mine. It was when she looked up and smiled at me I felt so convicted.

I have for many years been getting up every day at 3:00 a.m.; it's chronic pain that wakes me. Rather than focus on that, I decided years ago to get through it by praying, studying and reading my bible at that early hour. It's the best habit I've ever been drawn toward.

That morning was no different; I had already done my devotions prior to going to church. My conscience spoke to my heart after the little girl removed her coat and hung it on the back of her seat.

As she sat down she looked at me again and smiled the sweetest smile. The reflections of glitter from her dress seemed to dance around her face, which added a sparkling appearance to her pretty white teeth. However, I could detect the strong, unpleasant odor of cigarette smoke coming from her; she coughed again. Then again. *Maybe she's not sick but, instead, through no fault of her own, has had to inhale cigarette smoke! How sad.*

Poor little thing! If that's the case, she couldn't help it. Her little lungs had apparently been affected by someone smoking around her. Her body, hair and clothing reeked with the foul odor, but, unfortunately, because of the smell, it was difficult to see beyond my nose, through to my heart which, by this time, was heavy with compassion.

My eyes continued to observe her cuteness. She was wearing a pretty, black dress which glittered with sequins, and her long dark hair was neatly styled with braids, which had been meticulously woven close to her head. Her two siblings, who were wiggling around the mother, were just as cute and well dressed.

The toddler was a little boy with curly hair and he had on a black vest and black pants, topped off by a little red bow tie on a white shirt. On his feet were the cleanest, cutest, little brown suede boots. He kept his thumb in his mouth and, when he smiled at me, I could see deep dimples; he too had a terrible cough.

The infant had been wrapped in a blanket. When the blanket was removed, I could tell it was a baby girl. A sparkling white headband was around her black, curly hair and she had on a frilly red dress with white leggings and shiny, black, patent-leather shoes. I felt sadness when I observed the baby pushing her face to her mother's chest while trying to bring up the congestion rooted deeply in her lungs.

But one could easily see the mother had made sacrifices, which included letting her own self go so that her children would look good. She, too, had a vicious cough which was so recognizable. *I used to smoke, I knew that cough!* I could see no wedding ring on her finger, but her fingernails had been chewed to the quick. She looked very tired and had dark circles under her eyes, which occasionally glanced in my direction. Her hair was pulled back loosely into a ponytail, which rested in a hood that was attached to the dingy colored, thread-bare coat she wore.

It reminded me of the one time, I, too, had been a single mother sitting in church with my three little children and was caught up in an addiction. Even before that, I thought back to earlier days when I was just a little girl and remembered well how every adult in my life smoked. *I must have smelled that way, too!* It was normal back then and *obviously it's normal for her. Or is it?*

Perhaps I was wrong on all accounts, too judgmental, lacking in understanding. *Some of the odor may, indeed, be coming from cigarettes, but perhaps it is mixed with something else. I have known hardships. I, too, was once a single mother struggling and working long hours. But she has her kids in church; that is a good thing. She, like any good mother, may not look very put together, but her kids are. Maybe the only way they could get to church was to get a ride from someone who had a stinky car.*

The cough may, in fact, be from someone smoking, or, it's cold outside; maybe they live in a house with poor insulation or have to inhale fumes from a stove with inadequate ventilation just to keep warm, and the obnoxious odor permeating their clothing, skin and hair is from that house. I've had to live in those kinds of houses before. I don't know what struggles they are up against, but they are in the right place.

I can't take those negative thoughts back, but perhaps I can give them something. I smiled at all of them and was so thankful when the second hymn was sung and it came time to shake hands with the people around us. While gently squeezing the hand of the young mother, I looked into her hesitant eyes and reassuringly said to her, "Your children are beautiful and so are you."

Her little girl who was sitting next to me eagerly reached for my hand, as I did hers. I smiled, looked deeply into her eyes and said, "It's so nice to have you here today; I hope to see you again."

Father, forgive me. I pray they come back and I hope they again sit next to me. Lord, hear my prayer.

Author Interpretation:
Oh Lord, forgive me for what I say,
And for thoughts I think some days.
My mind often leads me astray;
Such a perfect person I'd be,
If my sins were washed away.
Who am I to judge, what people do
Each day of the year?
It's the good things people do

That others do not hear.
Such a beautiful world
In which we live.
<u>Understanding</u> is the key
And <u>what I need to give</u>.
(Written by: Kittye Sharron)

CHAPTER 11

My Red Pen Ministry

NOBODY ENJOYED SMOKING AS MUCH as I did and besides, back in the day, I was convinced I'd never be able to talk without a cigarette in my hand. (*As you can certainly see, I've managed quite well.*) I quit smoking in 1981 and, afterward, vowed I would be an instrument in sharing my success with others who had the same addiction. *Now, the first part of that last sentence said, "I quit" but I prefer using the wise words of my dear husband who states, "I have discovered anybody can quit. Instead, say, 'I don't smoke!' and mean it."*

I keep red pens with me at all times and whenever I see a person who is smoking alone, after a quick, silent prayer, I approach him/her and state, "I'm not selling anything; so may I give you something?"

"Are you crazy? Nothing in this world is free!"

"My gift is."

Most always anyone is willing to accept anything if it's free. When the person asks me what it is, I ask, "Have you ever tried quitting?"

Usual responses go something like, "Oh, I quit once, for 3 years!" OR, "I'll quit someday, but right now I'm having some issues." OR, "I've tried and can't do it."

I then hold up a red pen and say, "This is how I became a non-smoker over 35 years ago and, if you are interested, I'll tell you how I did it."

Usually, by that time, the person is inhaling a drag off his/her cigarette and blowing smoke in my face. That means, he/she is content and listening, so I continue.

I explain, "Whatever I was wearing I made sure it had pockets for I needed a handy place in which to keep a pen."

Raising the pen again, *I begin to demonstrate.*

"Quitting several habits is required, not just the inhaling of smoke. And when you stop one thing, you need to replace it with something else. That's where the pen comes in handy. One can hold it like a cigarette, put it between your fingers, between your lips, and make motions that would be indicative of flicking ashes off the end of it. There are even things you can do with this pen that you can't do with a lit cigarette! You can write or doodle with it! You can even suck on either end of it. *(I don't tell the person this, but it's like a pacifier; after all, isn't that why most people smoke, to pacify a need?")*

I continue…"You know, back in 1981, I didn't know the Lord but I had heard there was power in the name of Jesus. So, whenever I was tempted, I started whispering, "Jesus."

In conclusion, I say, "That method freed me up to be able to grab a pen instead of a cigarette. Oh sure, I was often tempted, but the longer I refrained from smoking, the easier it got. I discovered it was a whole lot cheaper than smoking, and a lot healthier! You really don't want to hear my medical history!"

Finally, before giving away the pen, I say, "When I decided to share my methods I chose red for the pen as a reminder of the color of the blood Jesus shed on the cross for my sins and yours. I don't know what your belief is, my friend, but I can tell you He hears our prayers, even when we just whisper His name."

I then give my new friend the pen and, before walking away, I say, "If this method works for you, I would like to ask a favor…please pass the idea on to someone else who may be struggling. By the way, what is your first name, I'd like to keep you in prayer." *After much practice, I've become pretty good at this praying thing!*

CHAPTER 12

Dancing with My Husband

"It's often been said that opposites attract. I agree. From early on, dancing was one of my desires. But until I met my dear husband, I never fully understood what it was all about. Now I have my own definition."

(QUOTE BY KITTYE SHARRON)

MY WONDERFUL HUSBAND, BILL, WAS born and raised in Muskegon, Michigan, *but I don't hold that against him!* You know, I could write an entire book on him alone. *He is the most amazing, compassionate, gentle, romantic individual I have ever known. I love him very much.*

Once our committed relationship began, he never ran away; he stuck by me through thick and thin…what a man! *He allows me freedom, encourages me when I'm down, comforts me when I cry, and pays more attention to me than I give him credit for.*

Bill is not 'hip' in his style of clothing. He loves his baggy blue jeans, but prides himself in wearing a nice shirt that matches the clothing I have on. It is he who tells me what color shirt he is wearing to church the following day. We have an understanding that it is up to me to make sure I wear something that will match the shirt he chose. *Our friends think I decide what we are wearing. (Best kept secrets!)*

As you may have already guessed, Bill is not extravagant and makes the best of everything. He has his own private library, his favorite place to read…sitting on the throne, *in the bathroom of our home!*

He inspires me. His love notes, often with innocently, misspelled words, *tickle me all the way to my toes!* Over the years, I have learned to decipher those notes and often chuckle at what they are written on (back of a paper plate, the roll of toilet tissue, bathroom mirror.) Or, he gets me the most beautiful card and doesn't remove the plastic wrapper before giving it to me. Once the laughter runs its course, the deep love is felt and I come to realize just how special he is. Many times, *every day*, there is a specific word that he says, just to me, which means, "I love you!" *How sweet is that?*

Sometimes, even his mistakes make me laugh, like the time he went to clean his glasses and grabbed the hair spray instead of the eyeglass cleaner. Most men, I suppose, would speak obscenities, but he can be heard saying, "Oh man!" *That's when you know he's made a blunder.* Or when he bypasses the instructions while assembling something and can't get it to work afterwards, he can be heard saying, "What idiot put this 'Mickey Mouse' thing together?"

Just yesterday, I heard him in the kitchen, "MAN!" When I asked him what had happened his response was, "I dropped my yogurt, twice!" The day before, he jumped up quickly from his chair, with clothes dripping wet. He had dosed off while holding a 16.9 ounce, uncapped bottle of water; need I say more?

It's important to Bill that we worship together and, when in church, he reaches for my hand to pray. During the service he is not ashamed to put his arm around me, often patting my shoulder or squeezing it gently. There are times he just holds my hand for no reason at all, and, *when we take a walk we do it holding hands.*

Once when I was teaching children in Sunday school, I looked up and there was my Bill holding the communion cup for me to be able to take communion. I thought it so sweet that he would think of me. For you see, it took extra effort for him to make his way down the long hall corridor *(he walks now with the aid of a cane.)*

Bill is a man of few words but, when he utters them, listen up! His spontaneous wit can be hilarious. Once he and I went to visit my relatives in Heber Springs, Arkansas, at the foothills of the Ozarks. During breakfast, while buttering his biscuit, my good ole Southern uncle, Melvin, asked my good ole 'Yankee' husband to pass him the sorghum molasses, but the funny part was the way in which he made his request.

In good ole' Southern drawl, Uncle Melvin said, "Bill, pass me 'them thar' sargums!"

Having no idea what he meant, Bill looked down at the things on the table and then up again and responded by asking, "How many of 'them thar sargums' are there?"

That same uncle while visiting at our house once asked Bill what kind of fish that was on our mantle. Bill's response, "A wooden one."

It's often been said that opposites attract. I agree. From early on, dancing was one of my desires. But until I met my dear husband, I never fully understood what it was all about. Now, I have my own definition.

Never, and I mean 'never', would Bill be caught dancing in public but, when we are alone and music is playing, he quite often slips his arm around my waist and leads me in what we call the "Bill-waltz." **And, of course, he would have a fit if I ever told anyone about it!**

I've come to realize what dancing is all about. It's following his lead to the beat of life's music. In order to hear that music, it's pertinent to study his moves and listen, not just with ears and eyes, but with the heart.

Keeping in step with the conversation shows respect; that's part of loving, following along and absorbing his words, laughing with him, whispering to each other, touching, while walking side by side. Our memories were made that way, and love grew by our recognizing the differences between us and accepting each other's imperfections.

Meals taste better when made with love. As a reminder of that, I keep a little spice can on the shelf next to my stove which says, "LOVE, Spice for Living."(I got it at my sister's yard sale years ago.) After cooking, I tell our children and grandchildren, "Well, I made it with love." Once, after I accidentally burned the pork chops, our little granddaughter said, "Nanny, I don't think you ought to make it with love anymore!"

Above my stove, treasured frames with "love" verses inside line the wall. Phrases include: 'Seasoned with love'; 'Welcome to Nanny's where all cupcakes are sprinkled with love'; 'Family is a little world created by love'; 'I love you'; 'May God's love surround you today and always'; Love bears all things, hopes all things, and endures all things. Love never fails (1 Corinthians: 13:8); 'The first rule of love is to listen'. It truly blesses my heart when our kids and grandchildren come to visit and stand around in the kitchen reading those sentiments.

Even though we said them to each other only twice upon a time, the vows Bill and I took, oh so long ago, were promises to love one another 'for better or for worse, for richer or for poorer, in sickness and in health, as long as we both shall live.' Those were both good and difficult words that were said before God and to each other as a covenant from our hearts. The meanings have blossomed and, with each passing year, our joint bond has strengthened.

At different times throughout our lives, life has brought us joy and life has brought us sorrow; we had seasons of plenty and have also been in want; we've been hurt and we've been healed, but we are in this marriage thing until we take our last breaths... Unlike society, we make our own music and develop our own dance; then we practice so as not to step on each other's toes.

Cute dance outfits left my heart's desire many years ago, and were replaced with touches of love... I can't even begin to count the number of times Bill has surprised me with cute, pretty things; before he will buy himself something, he makes sure to bring a gift home to me. By the way, it's not important to me anymore that I be a dancer, but a good partner, a helpmate, as we waltz through this life together.

> ### Author Interpretation:
> ### <u>SEASONS OF THE MIND</u>
> **The whisper of a summer's breeze holds a different secret for us all.**
> **Solemnly we may feel at ease, though there's a mystery as it calls.**
> **Yesterday the ground was frozen and, our hearts tried to melt the ice.**
> **Our memories returned to the summer again and, for a moment it was nice.**
> **And then the trees lost their leaves and everything seemed bare;**
> **Everything seemed stolen like the work of thieves, no one seemed to care.**
> **Then came the rain pouring down our face but, it was dried by the summer's breeze.**

It was warm and comforting like an embrace and, our minds were as still as the trees.
The answer lies in the sun that shines even though it may be covered by a cloud.
Some days things will seem to be fine but, nothing can be planted till the fields are plowed.
Then the seeds are covered and waiting to grow and, nature takes its course and already has assigned the ones that will survive the winds that blow
Only the strong will bloom in the seasons of the mind!
(Written by: Kittye Sharron in the 1970's)

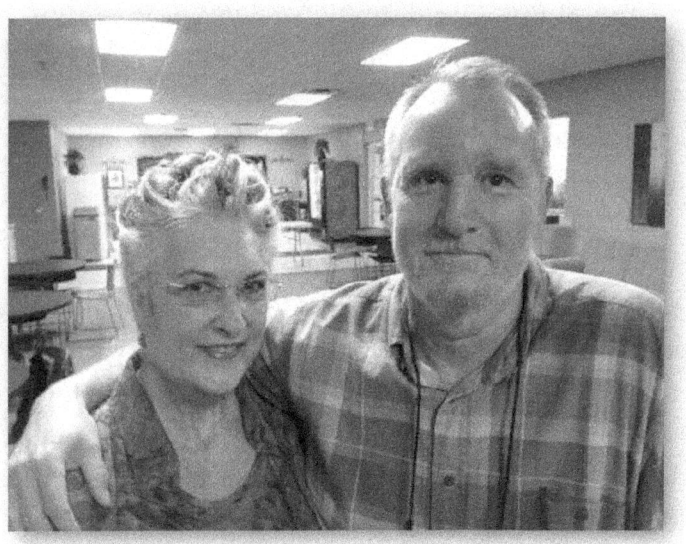

And that's how we got to this. We've come a long way... here we are in another season, our next chapter, my million dollar Bill & me (AKA Amy Kayleen).

CHAPTER 13

Parting Words

I HAVE BATTLED MANY HEALTH issues; however, through it all *I gained new insight into lifelong questions which I have attempted to weave throughout the chapters in this book. I'm grateful for another year in which to serve Him. Praise the One who gave me a new year of life...Jesus. For my future, I'm looking to Him, the author of all hope.*

Because of those health related bouts, I had to take a few detours in my writing, but *I'm back on track for now, another day in which to glorify Him.* Through all my cancers, not once did I lose my hair! Admittedly, there were a few times I doubted whether or not God had forgotten about me, but when I look back over the facts, I know without a doubt, He had me in the palm of His hand all along. He provided wisdom from above in countless ways. I'm convinced, He allowed me to go through these things in order to pass along some life-giving words in which to help my fellow man, my fellow sister. I pray that is what my story will do.

I know without a doubt that the bible is true and it says in Ecclesiastes 3:1-2 that there is a time for everything, a time to give birth and a time to die. All one has to do is look back in his/her own family to realize how true that is. Loved ones who have gone before us, even our animals (*our Dixie girl and Biscuit boy are both gone, too,*) but, for today, I live. However, death to our body is part of life and, if you think about it, we spend our entire lives preparing to meet our Maker, not in body, but in spirit. None of us will escape; *it's a sure thing.* Our souls, we all have them, are the parts in us that will live on after the vessels carrying them die. They will go to Heaven or Hell; the choice is ours.

Future treatment of my condition includes undergoing frequent cancer screenings. In order to detect any growths or areas of concern before it's too late, preventative testing will include regular visits to my physicians, CT and/or MRI scans, diagnostic x-rays, and bloodwork.

Serious medical problems have plagued me since I was born and the way I got through them was *to get through them.* My passionate desire is to avail myself in helping others who are sincere, but discouraged, to find healing, gain insight, and take heart so they can live out their faith with courageous compassion. Here are some of the methods I have used, *and will continue to use,* along with some of my favorite things:

1) Give all glory to God, He is the one I cried out to time after time. It wasn't by chance prayers were answered. *Divine intervention took place and the world needs to know how it came about.*
2) I heard a faithful man say this once and I think there is some truth to it. "If the only time I talk to the Lord is during a crisis, then He may just keep me in a crisis situation; He wants to hear from me." *I get it, Lord, I really get it!*
3) 1 Corinthians 1:25-31 speaks volumes to my heart. It tells me that though I am a frail, weak vessel, God can use me. *But I have to be willing*; for the will of God is found in the path of obedience. James 4:8a says: "Draw near to God and He will draw near to you." *(I love that!)*
4) Find the simple things in life and enjoy them. What you are tomorrow, you are becoming today. *Yes, yes today will be yesterday tomorrow.* Are you using all your resources? When you find them, follow this basic rule: keep yourself pure. (1 Thessalonians 4:1-12)
5) Freshly laundered sheets, which have been dried on a clothesline, have a sweet, clean fragrance. So does God's word. *It washes my mind, renews my spirit, cleanses my heart and is medicine for my soul.* (Apply

liberally, experience healing.) Get in the Word, stay in the Word and *find out how He wants me to live. I should never rely only on my own understanding.*

6) A good reason for putting together a photo album of my honey and me: so I can fall in love all over again.

7) Thrift store and garage sale items are inexpensive and typically have already been broken in! Usually clothes have gone through the wash at least once, which is an added bonus… they won't fade as do new ones.

8) Have faith in God. It means you have peace even when you don't have all the answers. My minister said to look at science through the lens of God. If the Bible says it, believe it. *That works for me!*

9) Give to others what we ourselves desperately crave. *I desired knowledge of my medical mysteries; therefore, I have shared my journey with you. Knowledge is a great thing to have and even when you give it away, you still have it. Besides, as the old song says, 'this world is not my home; I'm just passing through' and as I stroll my prayer is that whatever I do, whatever I say while I'm here, will be pleasing to my Father in Heaven, the Lord my God.*

10) Move forward; keep going in a new way. I heard someone say to build bridges, not walls. *I think that is the Christian way of doing things.*

11) My son preached a sermon once saying, "Sin will take you further than you wanted to go; it will keep you longer than you wanted to stay; and will cost you more than you wanted to pay." *That's been my experience!*

12) Listen to your body and, if it tells you there is a problem, more than likely there is. Just because one doctor has no solution, never be afraid to seek a second opinion, even a third, or all the way to twenty one or more. *Persistence saved my life!* Your life counts for something. It may just be that the Lord wants to use you for His glory! He is the Great Physician, the author of all hope and He puts people in our lives to do His bidding.

13) *I'm probably addicted to writing, but I don't believe that's a bad thing; just as long as I'm spending time with God.* Writing is a good way to get things out, it's very therapeutic and, as a writer friend of mine said, "It's like washing yuck off dishes!"

14) My sister reminded me not to borrow trouble from tomorrow; there is this day to get through first. *Robyn Louise is pretty smart!*

15) I gain strength when others are praying for me. Therefore, I try to return the favor as often as I can.

16) Healthy is a very good word. *I also like the words benign, non-cancerous or not malignant.* It's great to be alive, sane and in remission. My helpful hints for

staying healthy include: sunshine, fresh air, exercise, water, Mediterranean-type diet, rest and laughter.

17) I recently read a sign that said, "Happiness for Marriage: When you are wrong, admit it; when you are right, shut up!" *Tried and true!*

18) If you have never placed your faith in Jesus, there is no better time than now. Perhaps you would like to open your bible and follow along:

(Romans 1:16 ~ God's promise for salvation is for everyone; it comes only from God.

Ephesians 2:8-9 ~ we cannot do anything to earn salvation; it is a free gift.

Romans 3:23 ~ Sin separates all people from God. No matter how good we think we are, we cannot measure up to God's standard.

Romans 6:23 ~ Sin causes eternal death. God allows each person to choose whether to accept or reject Christ. All who reject Him will spend eternity in Hell.

John 1:1 ~ Jesus is God, but He became human for us.

Romans 5:8 ~ God loves each person. He does not like sin, but He loves the sinner. He loved us so much, He gave His only Son to die for our sins. We should have died.

Acts 3:19 ~ Repentance is turning away from our sins and turning to God in faith.

Romans 10:9&13 ~ all people are asked to confess that they are sinners; then to place their faith in Jesus by placing their lives in His hands and asking Him to lead.

Have you placed your faith in Jesus and asked Him into your life? Would you like to, now? In case you are lost and going in the wrong direction, *like I was, here's what I did:*

Just whisper…, "Jesus"; talk to Him, confess your sins, and ask for His forgiveness. Turn from your sins and turn to God. Invite Him into your life. Then get yourself into a bible-believing church. If you don't know what to do next, humble yourself; tell someone there that you only just arrived and need some instruction. Then start listening to the songs and the Word as it is preached. Enjoy the dance you'll feel in your heart, for if you believe that which scripture reveals, you will know a better home awaits, and you have a holy partner who will promenade you into glory.

Author's Final Note:
There will come a day,
When my voice will be no more.
So I leave behind these parting words.
The end will <u>not</u> come
When the dance is done, for I believe,
Life then, will have just begun.
(Written by: Kittye Sharron)

(*NOTE: Chapters 14 & 15 includes hairstyle tips and various pictures. The ending of this book will direct you to my website and, my YouTube channel, where you can view the 'how-to-do-it-yourself' video for mastering the hairstyle featured on the front cover.)

It is finished ...but don't stop reading! (Concluded in Epilogue.)

CHAPTER 14

Let's Talk Hair & Gray & Izzy!

*I'd rather people say, "She's too young to be gray!"
than to say, "She's too old to be coloring her hair!"*

(QUOTE BY: KITTYE SHARRON)

DOWN THROUGH THE YEARS I'VE had many hairstyles and various colors; (i.e. dark braids, short with blondish streaks, pixie styled, long, curled, straight, up in a ponytail, etc.) The following pages will show pictures of a few of those coiffures. The hairstyle pictured on the front cover of this book (and at the end of this chapter) has served me well since I made the decision to put the peroxide and color back in the box and go with the crown of age. It was either that or pluck out all my eyebrows and eyelashes, for they too, along with the roots on my head, were beginning to turn white. Scripture helped me to make the decision to embrace the inevitable.

"A gray head is a crown of glory; it is found in the way of righteousness." (Proverbs 16:31)

I started beauty school when I was an immature sixteen year old. Funny, I completed it but never went to get my license because at the time I decided I didn't want to work around women all day. (Then, when I become an Executive Housekeeper I had a staff of 55+ workers, mostly women. *Go figure!) I often think back to one of my early days of styling hair and other than a good laugh, it didn't have a very good ending.*

Robyn's best friend in high school was Isabelle (whom we nicknamed Izzy.) Izzy was like one of the family and was at our house more than at her own. She stood not even 5 feet tall and was cute as a bug's ear. That is, until I almost burned off her bangs!

In the 60's, curling irons had become quite the craze; but back then they had only one setting…hot. I needed the practice for my beauty school training, so Izzy let me use the ceramic coated, skinny barreled curling iron on her bangs. Not knowing how long to leave it on her hair, when smoke began swirling around her head, that's when I figured it had been on long enough. When I unrolled the tight clamp, I was shocked. Her bangs were curled so tightly she looked like a funky little poodle! When she looked in the mirror, her eyes got so wide, I thought they would jump out of their sockets. She immediately began trying to comb her bangs to straighten them, but it made no difference…boing…the curl was too tight.

To make matters worse, I jokingly told Izzy it was going to stay that way until it grew out; she wasn't amused. It took soaking her entire head with water in order to relax the tight curl. After that, she never would allow me to touch her hair! *Imagine that!*

So, as you can see, I haven't always been the best when it comes to a hairstyle. It took many years of trial and error, I can now fast forward to this era. I no longer use a curling iron. I have set aside this chapter to share some techniques/tips that work well for me. They include:

1) Embrace who God made you to be. I had my day, yesterday is gone, and *today I am gray, it's the season!*
2) Wash your hair at least twice a week, if not more. It is said, "Cleanliness is next to godliness" (2 Corinthian's 7:1b "Let us cleanse ourselves...")
3) After washing the hair, comb, not brush, all the snarls out of the wet hair. *(I found that brushing my hair when wet caused broken ends.)*
4) For this hairstyle, when necessary, cut/trim the hair on your head while the hair is wet, using a razor, not scissors. Otherwise, the ends will be too blunt; you want your curls to smooth out nicely without springing up. To achieve that, regardless of how thick your hair is, never allow anyone to thin it. Doing so will cause "twigs of hair" to stick out from the rolls (you don't want that.)

5) After washing, dry the hair. (This is the relaxing part…) Lay down on your back with your head slightly off the edge of the bed. Using the blow dryer, dry your hair until it is not quite dry, rather leave it a little damp. (*I often close my eyes while doing this, breathe deeply, let it out slowly, and thank the Lord for what He has done.*)
6) Every morning, while standing, bow your head down and, starting from the back of your neckline, brush your hair forward. (*While doing so, that is a good time to whisper a 'thank-you' to the Lord for a good night's sleep*); then take a small section of hair at the front of your hairline and slowly raise your head up. Braid that which you are holding, I call it, 'Making a God Knot'. (*In reference to Ecclesiastes 4:12: "A cord of 3 strands is not quickly torn apart."*) That one section you have braided is the foundation for the hairstyle. (*Think of it as the rock…a firm foundation.*) Wrap loose ends around it and roll that downward in the direction of your back, secure with a long bobby pin. Take the section of hair next to it and roll it toward the braided knot; secure with bobby pin. Repeat for the rest of your hair. (See tips below.)
7) Every night, take the pins out and let your hair down. Bow your head and brush your hair from the back of the neckline. (*While in that position, with your head down, close your eyes and pray. Thank God for another*

day.) Your hair will have a lot of body to it, like you have just taken out rollers; it will look great. Smile, wash your face, and brush your teeth. Smile again. Go and kiss your husband and say, "Honey, I'm ready for bed!"

8) **TIP:** It's helpful to be able to see the back of your head while styling your hair. In order to do that, you may want to affix a long mirror to the wall in your bedroom (or wherever you do your hair). Do this by first attaching short chains to the mirror, which will make it easier to slant downward. It's also helpful, while styling, to have a standing mirror on a side table with which to view your profile. *(It is easier for me to sit on a stool while doing up my hair, so my mirror is at a height to allow for that.)*

9) **TIP:** Never open the bobby pin with your teeth; instead get accustomed to opening it with your forefinger. *(Save the teeth!) If your hair is thin or, you need extra support or, if there is a problem area, hair pins can be inserted.*

10) **TIP**: It is suggested to use long bobby pins to secure the curls. (You can find them at the Beauty Supply in different colors; *I use gray and black to blend with my hair.)*

11) **TIP**: I use small couture clips for added definition around the edges of my hair, or anywhere I want to

create a greater, darker space between the curls; also they add a little bling.

12) **TIP:** In order to establish depth for each curl, **start pinning the bobby pin in the curl next to it.** (Demonstrated in the online video.)

13) **TIP:** After your hair is in place, spray with a dry, brushable styling hairspray - not one that is stiff. You want to be able to brush your hair each night without having a stiff residue. Follow-up with a light spritz of weightless shine spray.

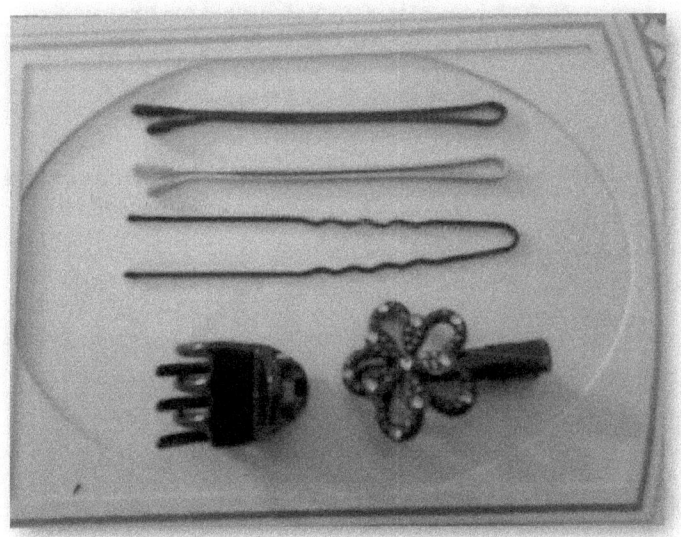

Long bobby pins in two colors to match my hair; hairpin and clips (as per tips #9, #10 & #11).

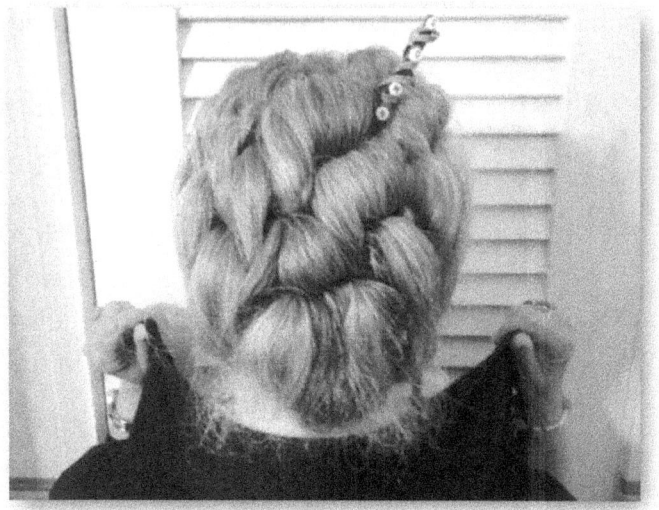

Back of my hair.

Hairstyle by Kittye Sharron with handmade SDHB hair stick.
It's all in my head!

CHAPTER 15

Pictures & Years of Hairstyles

Excerpt from The Longest Letter: Incredible Hope: *"I was just a little girl from Arkansas who answered to the name of Amy Kayleen."*

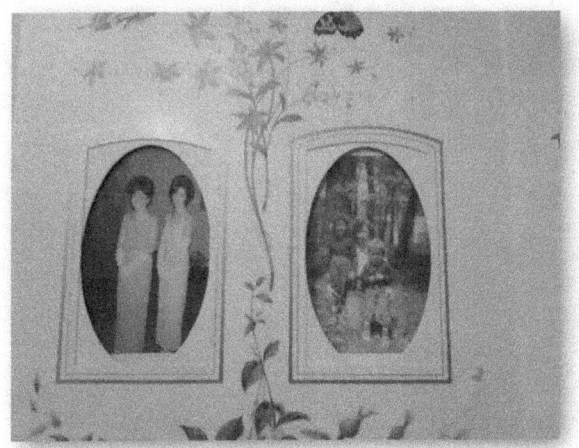

Picture on the left: High school prom (sisters: left to right: AKA Robyn Louise & Amy Kayleen.)

Picture on the right: Early days (left to right: AKA Amy Kayleen, Mother/Peggy Marie, and Robyn Louise.)

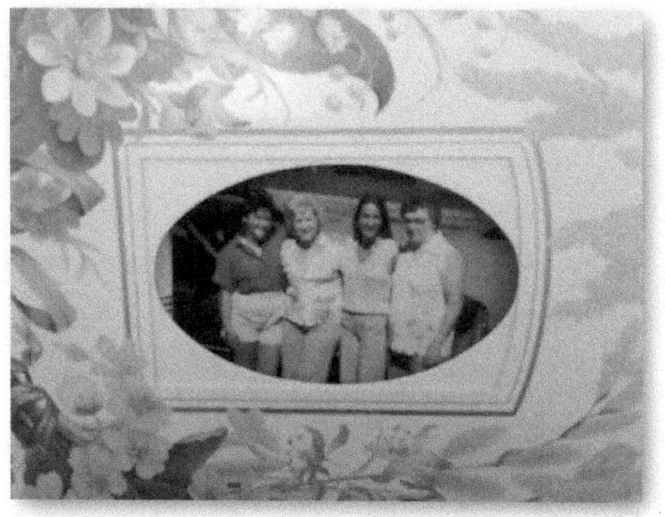

Left to right: AKA Robyn Louise, Mother (Peggy Marie), Amy Kayleen, and Mama (1983).

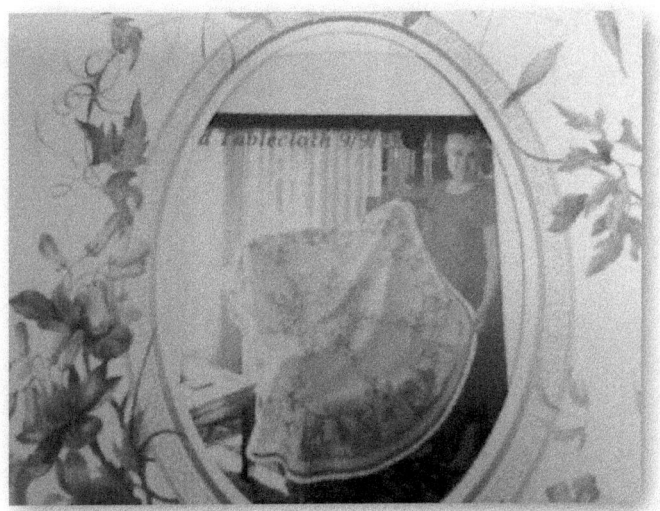

Me (Aka Amy Kayleen), showing finished, embroidered yellow tablecloth which took 24 years to complete.

Excerpt from The Longest Letter: Incredible Hope ~ "I'll finish that tablecloth someday in her honor. It will be a beautifully unique tapestry, woven with threads of many colors, and like her, will always hold a special place in the garden of my heart."

EPILOGUE (2017)

Oh no, another abnormal mammogram! And if that wasn't bad enough, a recent CT scan showed a suspicious growth on my remaining kidney. Worry x 2.

In order for my Spectrum oncologist, Doctor Melnik, to take a closer look at what was going on with my breasts, a diagnostic mammogram was ordered along with an ultrasound. The test results revealed fibrous tissue and even though there was evidence of some small cysts, nothing vascular showed; they don't pose a threat. Just to be sure, the recommendation was made for a repeat of those tests in 6 months and they will watch for any changes. Whew! *But I'm not out of the woods, yet!*

I prayed, "Lord, what about my one and only left kidney? The last CT scan showed a growth on it and I'm due to be seen by the urologist. However, my previous doctor moved out of state. What do I do now?"

Personally, I've had a difficult time finding specialists in this area who are knowledgeable about the SDHB gene mutation. I remembered how impressed I was with my sister's urologist. Last year she, too, had a growth on her kidney and was seen by a Spectrum Urologist, Dr. Brian Lane. He had researched SDHB and knew exactly what to do. Quick action to remove the growth probably saved her life, for afterward, the biopsy showed it had been cancerous. *He is familiar with our family history. I need to see him!*

The distance between Muskegon and Grand Rapids was approximately 45 miles, but it was worth the trip. With bated breath, I watched the face of Dr. Lane as he reviewed my previous CT and MRI's. Relief followed as I heard him say that because there were no changes and he could see nothing vascular, it appeared the cyst on my one and only kidney was harmless. (*I have a new favorite word, harmless!*) Just to be sure, he ordered another preventative CT scan and bloodwork. The final result confirmed there was nothing vascular, no change from prior scan, nothing to worry about. *I'm in good hands!*

I guess I feel as though Dr. Lane, as well as Dr. Melnik, Dr. Ogas, Dr. Hiemenga, Dr. Lomeo and other doctors who are on my care team, impress me with their running "toward" a problem rather than "away" from it. They desire to be part of the solution and, for that, I am grateful.

And so, my friend, I leave you with this...

I may not have gotten ole' Bernard the Brute's autograph when I was a little girl; but *it's okay*. What would I have done with it, anyway? The experience actually served me better just using it as an illustration to include in my life story. Besides, why did I think I needed an old wrestler's signature?

My hairstyle has become my autograph... I view my genetic makeup as the fingerprint of God, a way in which to glorify Him. Because, you see, there are others who have similar, rare circumstances, and may be struggling with preposterous symptoms related to SDHB or other complicated issues. *I had you in mind when I wrote my story. I trust my signature will serve you well. (Follow the links below to view the "how-to-do-it-yourself" hairstyle video.)* (***Read just two more sentences!**)

THE END

*Final Note: I have been given the desires of my heart. *Now, each and every day is a precious gift.*
(***A special message to the reader appears in Acknowledgements.)**
Lord bless your home.
By: KITTYE SHARRON
The hairstyle video is on my website @ www.kittyesharron.com ; it's also on my YouTube channel @ https://youtu.be/rAEK:3GgfsQ (Kittye Sharron-It's All in Your Head Hair Tutorial.)
Following are: Acknowledgements, websites, and Author page.

ACKNOWLEDGEMENTS

Bill ~ my loyal husband and best friend ~ thank you for your love, patience and tolerance during the many hours I spent ignoring you while putting together, first "The Longest Letter: Incredible Hope"; then (less than a year later,) "It's All in Your Head! The Gene that Stumped the Doctors." You're the best for always standing by my side, holding my hand and cheering me on during my meltdowns. It was a huge undertaking when you asked me to be your wife, taking into account I had 3 children, but loving them and me. You had no idea you were getting a 'scratch and dent' model! (Thanks for keeping me.)

My mother ~ (AKA Peggy Marie) thank you for shedding blood to bring me into the world and your inspiration along life's journey. The sacrifices you have always made for me will forever be ingrained in my heart. You are a great blessing. *I love you, Mother.*

My children ~ thank you for loving me, in spite of all the mistakes I made. Also, for calling me "Mom", encouraging me, and joining my online pages. Oh, how I love you all.

My grandchildren ~ thank you, "*little darlins,*" for calling me Nanny, listening to the stories I have written, and telling me you liked them. Has anybody told you yet today that you are loved? *I love you.*

My sister (AKA Robyn Louise) God knew I needed a sister, you were the best choice; I couldn't have asked for a better one. You and I have carved a pathway for which we knew not the way but, by the grace of God we are alive, and I'm so thankful I had you to walk beside me. Thank you for reviewing my manuscript, if it gets by your beautiful eyes, I won't have a thing to worry about. Please be advised, if there are any of my famous, dangling participles in the book, it's not your fault; I snuck a few sentences in without your review! *(I love Ernie's description of us, "The scratch and dent sisters!")*

Kerry Lee Westveld – Thank you for reviewing my manuscript, doing my photo shoot and, for designing the awesome book cover of, "It's All in Your Head! The Gene That Stumped the Doctors." Your skill and professionalism really show through in your creativity; you are an amazing perfectionist. I would recommend anyone looking for an excellent photographer to contact you @ www.kerryleephotography.

Katherine Averill – Thank you for sharing your time, effort, and expertise in video- graphing the "It's All in Your Head" video. You did a great job and I appreciate it so much.

Ashley Haveman Gabrielse – Thank you, my friend, for meeting with me numerous times and sharing your knowledge of the computer. I couldn't have done it without your help.

Dr. Carl A. Ogas, M.D., Seminole Shores Internal Medicine, PC (Muskegon, MI) ~ My primary physician, I thank you for taking a genuine interest in my not-so-ordinary set of circumstances; and for prompting me to push my family toward testing. Your attention to detail is very noticeable and most appreciated.

Dr. Paul Lomeo, D.O., Shoreline ENT., PLC (Muskegon, MI) ~ Thank you for providing me with your expert care and for allowing God to work through your healing hands to mend my body. On more than one occasion you found the problem and knew exactly what to do.

Dr. Marianne Melnik, MD, FACS Surgical Oncologist/Breast Surgeon, Lemmen-Holton Cancer Pavilion/Spectrum (Grand Rapids, MI) ~ I prayed for a miracle doctor and God sent you. You, then, steered me in the direction I should go. I'll be forever indebted for your wisdom and dedication to your patients. You are terrific.

Dr. Judith Hiemenga, MD Clinical Geneticist and, Mary Mobley, MEd, MS, CGC Genetic Counselor, Lemmen-Holton Cancer Pavilion/Spectrum (Grand Rapids, MI) – Together you two ladies put my mind at ease, never once questioning my sanity; bless your little hearts. Thank you for being interested and caring enough to find answers for my lifelong dilemma. Your combined efforts and knowledge of genetic testing probably saved my life and several of my family members.

Dr. Brian R. Lane, MD, PhD Division Chief, Urology @ Lemmen-Holton Cancer Pavilion/Spectrum (Grand Rapids, MI) – Thank you for all the research you have done, and continue doing, regarding SDHB. You proved yourself worthy of my respect when treating my sister; *and now, your willingness to be my urologist, too, is greatly appreciated. We are in good hands.*

My friends ~ you know who you are. In the book, your names may have been changed, but you will recognize yourselves. I'll be eternally grateful for the friendship role you have played in my life.

All my Facebook contacts ~ thank you for "Liking" me, especially those of you who follow my Facebook, Kittye Sharron Author Page. Your involvement has given me courage and boosted my confidence.

Alexandra Wisen, Photographer ~ thank you for taking the beautiful rainbow photograph, (2013,) and so graciously donating it for the cover of my first published book, "The Longest Letter: Incredible Hope." (It is also featured in the 4th chapter of this book.) Website: www.alexandrawisen.com/

Create Space ~ Once again, it was a wonderful experience working with your expert staff. Thank you for the helpful guidance you provided during the publishing process.

*To the reader ~ Special message: Thank you for taking the time to read this. My hope is that you have enjoyed the book. Please take a moment now and rate: "It's All in Your Head! The Gene that Stumped the Doctors." (**5 * *would thrill me!***) Your voice is very important to me; you may want to contact me just to say hello, or, if you have had a similar medical experience, feel free to share your story with me. (Without someone to talk to, it can be a lonely world.) Furthermore, I would love to read an honest review, from special you, with just a few short sentences stating what you liked about the book and why; or didn't like and why. If you are on Facebook and want to join my author page, come and "Like" me @ https://www.facebook.com/KittyeSharron. Visit my website @ www.kittyesharron.com and say hello to me on my YouTube channel @ https://youtu.be/rAEK:3GgfsQ your feedback will be greatly appreciated. Thank you.

Lord bless your home.

KITTYE SHARRON (also known as: Amy Kayleen)

IT'S ALL IN YOUR HEAD! THE GENE THAT STUMPED THE DOCTORS.

ABOUT THE AUTHOR

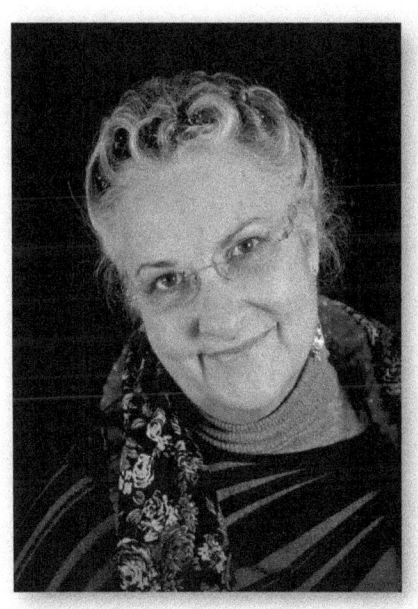

KITTYE SHARRON SAYS SHE COMES from very humble beginnings and is most grateful for that. She states, "I've been transplanted from the cotton fields of Arkansas, transferred to the fruit orchards of Michigan, and transformed by the journey! It's what made me who I am today, and I'm a survivor!"

Her journey began in 1948. Raised by a single, divorced mother, Kittye Sharron survived childhood sexual abuse and divorce, Pheochromocytoma disease, thyroid cancer, breast cancer, kidney cancer, and Post Traumatic Stress Disorder, just to name a few. Those are some of the topics she writes about.

She began studying in the Criminal Justice field and ended up making a career in Florida as a Registered Executive Housekeeper (R.E.H.) Also, she taught the Executive Housekeeping curriculum.

She says, "I wore many hats along the way."

Now retired, she and her husband reside in Muskegon, Michigan. She is often asked to speak at various groups and give her testimony. Her writing includes children's stories and poems. She began writing her first book, *The Longest Letter: Incredible Hope* in 1988 and published it in April, 2016. Her current book titled: *It's All in Your Head! The Gene That Stumped the Doctors*, has been being compiled since 1974.

Kittye Sharron has a goal! It is to present her work in a way that targets hurting people who are barely hanging on to the threads of Christianity. Her desire is to reach an audience for whom hope is difficult to grasp because something, or someone they love and care for, is sucking the very life out of them! Her aim is to provide clarity and a way to escape the throes of a sinful world by providing personal solutions toward victory.

www.ingramcontent.com/pod-product-compliance
Lightning Source LLC
Chambersburg PA
CBHW071428180526
45170CB00001B/261